Colonoscopy
**Diagnosis and Treatment
of Colonic Diseases**

Colonoscopy

Diagnosis and Treatment of Colonic Diseases

HIROMI SHINYA, M.D.

Chief of Surgical Endoscopy Unit
Beth Israel Medical Center, New York

Clinical Professor of Surgery
Mount Sinai School of Medicine, New York

IGAKU-SHOIN   New York · Tokyo

Published and distributed by

IGAKU-SHOIN Ltd.,
5-24-3 Hongo, Bunkyo-ku, Tokyo

IGAKU-SHOIN Medical Publishers, Inc.,
1140 Avenue of the Americas, New York, N.Y. 10036

Library of Congress Cataloging in Publication Data

Shinya, Hiromi.
  Colonoscopy, diagnosis and treatment of colonic diseases.

  Bibliography: p.
  Includes index.
  1. Colonoscopy. I. Title. [DNLM: 1. Colonic diseases. 2. Colonoscopy. WI 520 S556c]
RC804.C64S47   616.3′4   81-6697
                                   AACR2

ISBN: 0-89640-065-4

Printed and bound in U.S.A.

10 9 8 7 6 5 4 3 2

Preface

Colonoscopy is a well-established diagnostic and therapeutic procedure. Nonetheless, few comprehensive textbooks on colonoscopy provide guidance for beginners as well as advanced refinements in technique for experts. The need for such a book has been suggested and impressed upon me by many physicians visiting our endoscopy unit. The one-man technique, which was devised by our unit, is not usually taught in endoscopy and gastroenterology programs. The two-man technique is more commonly used worldwide. I believe that the latter technique is less efficient and allows less than total control of the instrument by the endoscopist. My credo is that the endoscope is literally an extension of the endoscopist; both components should function as a smooth working unit.

This book has been prepared to provide a step-by-step description of what I believe are the proper colonoscopic techniques. Although experience is truly the best teacher, guidelines must be set to properly acquire that experience. An attempt has been made to provide such guidelines and coverage in this book to help develop and improve colonoscopy and polypectomy skills. In addition, illustrations show the endoscopic appearances of diseases of the colon to help identify and characterize what the instrument visualizes or removes.

I have performed approximately 45,000 colonoscopies and more than 10,000 polypectomies for various lesions larger than 0.5 cm in diameter. This book shares with readers the lessons that I have learned so that others can avoid the pitfalls and frustrations they might otherwise experience in the course of acquiring expertise.

Furthermore, if the technique is standardized and carefully executed, patient care will be improved. I have endeavored to describe my methods clearly and illustrate them well so that colonoscopists with any degree of experience may benefit.

My interest in endoscopy and colonoscopy began when I was a resident in 1967. At that time, I perceived some of the applications of the technique, but I have been gratified that its scope and horizon have been expanded beyond my expectations.

    That this book has been transformed from a personal dream to a publication that almost did not reach fruition is due in great part to the encouragement (and occasional nagging) of the publishers. Without the endoscopy staff of Beth Israel Hospital and my office staff, I would have had neither the time nor the energy to complete this book. My heartfelt thanks go to Dr. Ken Mori, pathologist, and Dr. Mark Cwern for the many hours that they spent reviewing the manuscript; to my fellows, Dr. Robyn Karlstadt and Dr. Gary Wolf, for providing the stimulus to answer and think through answers to their basic queries; and to all my colleagues, who continue to refine our knowledge in this ever-burgeoning field. I thank those who helped me write in the English language, which is not my native tongue. I thank Rona Schorr for long hours spent typing and retyping each draft. And last, but certainly not least, I extend my gratitude to my family for their patience during the many hours it took to develop and write this book.

Hiromi Shinya, M.D.

Contents

    (ADENOMAS) SHOWING MALIGNANT
    DEGENERATION   195

17. COMPLICATIONS: PREVENTION AND
    MANAGEMENT   199

    Diagnostic Colonoscopy   199

    Biopsy   202

    Colonoscopic Polypectomy   202

18. FOLLOW-UP EXAMINATION   209

19. SPECIAL APPLICATIONS OF
    COLONOSCOPY   211

    BIBLIOGRAPHY   218

    INDEX   229

Colonoscopy
**Diagnosis and Treatment
of Colonic Diseases**

1

Introduction

Fiberoptic instruments have revolutionized the diagnosis and treatment of colonic disease, especially in the early detection of carcinoma. Because of the advantages of direct visualization, the fiberoptic colonscope is an advance over the rigid sigmoidoscope: it allows greater depth of insertion, and it provides the capability to maneuver around and through narrowed and angulated areas. Early identification of malignant and premalignant lesions with this diagnostic technique affords, in theory, a higher cure rate since lesions may be recognized earlier after initial appearance, before detection by barium roentgenograms and before metastases have developed. Furthermore, prophylactic removal of premalignant polypoid lesions may lower the incidence and prevent the development of malignant disease. Although colonoscopy is obviously superior to sigmoidoscopy for thorough evaluation of the rectum and colon, its use requires greater expertise and training. Nonetheless the beneficial effects of the procedure are widely recognized by clinicians in all specialties. A vigorous program to detect and remove polyps to prevent carcinoma of the colon is merely an extension of the same principle advocated by Gilbertson and co-workers and applied to rectal carcinoma 15 years ago.

HISTORY

Endoscopy can be traced to early civilization. Ancient Greeks were aware of this type of examination, as evidenced by Hippocrates' description of the rectal speculum in a treatise on fistulae. More recently, in 1853, Desormeaux described an instrument for the examination of the anus and rectum. Kelly, of Baltimore, has been responsible for major advances in the utilization and design of the sigmoidoscope.

Rigid sigmoidoscopy is an integral part of a complete examination. It is unnecessary to enumerate the benefits this diagnostic tool has conferred upon all physicians in their diagnostic testing. Unfortunately, however, most physicians fail to examine completely the distal sigmoid area, 25 cm from the anal verge. Furthermore, recent studies have shown a changing pattern of the dis-

1

tribution of diseases, particularly cancer, with a proximal shift of lesions, making the need for colonoscopy important.

The principle of transmitting light waves and optical images along coated glass and plastic fibers was described in 1870 and applied initially in an industrial setting, in 1951. In 1958, Hirschowitz et al described the "fiberscope," which was a flexible instrument that could be advanced into the stomach and duodenum. Later reports described in vivo characteristics of normal and abnormal stomach and duodenal mucosa. Further advances produced technically superior instruments that are constantly being refined, even today.

The principle of the fiberoptic method is based on total internal reflection. This phenomenon occurs when light at certain angles strikes an interface between a substance that has a high refractive index (e.g., glass) and one that has a low refractive index (for example, air or a coating on the glass). Light enters one end of the cylindric rod and strikes the surface at an angle greater than the critical angle required for total internal reflection. The light then advances longitudinally by a series of internal reflections and exits at the other end of the rod, even if acutely bent. Thus, transmission of light through fiberoptic rods is superior to that through other optical equipment, such as lenses and mirrors. The fine glass or plastic rods are coated with an extraordinarily thin coating of low refractive material and then drawn into bundles. Each fiber (or rod) must be placed to occupy the same relative position at both ends of the bundle, so that the image of the illuminated surface can be transmitted exactly as it appears to the eye. In modern instruments, the fiber bundle contains approximately 30,000 fine coated glass fibers, providing fine resolution and an accurate picture of the observed surface. The transmitted light is "cold," and this feature eliminates the potential problem of raising the internal temperature of the human body.

Needless to say, the development of this instrument and its advantages of flexibility, accurate representation of a projected image and bright transillumination presaged a new era for gastrointestinal diagnosis and management.

The Japanese led progress in this "endoscopic era" by making technical improvements in the instrument and by popularizing it. Because of the high incidence of gastric carcinoma in Japan, early efforts were directed toward upper gastrointestinal endoscopy. Especially notable in this area was the development of the gastrocamera, which could be introduced to photograph the interior of the viscera. Modifications of the gastroscope permitted greater flexibility, including the ability to "retroflex" in the stomach and visualize the cardia from below, and improve the visual capability for complete examination.

Colonoscopy was still in its infancy in Japan, probably due to the lower incidence of colorectal disease in the East. Oshiba and Watanabe, Niwa et al, and Kanazawa and Tanaka attempted to apply the principles of gastroscopy to an instrument that could be used to examine the colon but were unable to develop one that advanced beyond the sigmoid colon. In the United States, Turrell, in 1963 and 1967, also reported difficulty in advancing the flexible scope beyond the proximal sigmoid colon. In 1969, Overholt demonstrated that a scope could be advanced to the proximal sigmoid and descending colon. In England, Dean and Shearman and Fox reported similar results at this time. In 1969, we attempted to evaluate the possibility of complete colon examination using a fiberoptic colonoscope. With fluoroscopic control to guide our initial efforts, we were able to perform more than 100 examinations, and there were no complications. With increasing skill and experience, we developed a longer colono-scope for examination to the ileocecal valve and, in some cases, the terminal ileum and were able to restrict the use of fluoroscopy for occasional difficult cases.

Furthermore, in September 1969 we initiated attempts to remove polyps through the colonoscope with the use of an electro-surgical unit. The same technique was also applied to polyps in the stomach. This approach eliminated the need for laparotomy, and its attendant morbidity and mortality, and elimi-nated situations where a polyp was missed. We reported the technique of endo-scopic polypectomy for the first time to the American Society of Gastroin-testinal Endoscopy in May, 1971. We performed colonoscopy without the use of complicated and cumbersome maneuvers, such as passage of a string through the mouth to the anus for retrograde guidance of the colonoscope, as described by Provenzale and Ravignos and Hiratsuka. Reliance on these methods would probably have slowed subsequent advancements.

By June 1971, our experience in performing 410 colonoscopies without com-plications was reported. At the time of this writing, we have carried out more than 45,000 colonoscopies with few complications and no deaths.

Recent developments have included improvements in instrument design that have made it safer and easier to use. Because of the technique's worldwide popularity as well as adequate education and training of hospital staff, co-lonoscopy now benefits patients without exposing them to unnecessary hazards.

Late in 1969, after gaining experience and establishing confidence with the technique, we explored the therapeutic possibilities of the instrument. Initially, we removed pedunculated polyps using a home-made snare and standard elec-trocautery unit at all levels of the colon. We next excised some sessile polyps with few complications and no mortality. At that time, we also fulgurated small polyps (less than 0.5 cm in length) after biopsy or totally removed them by biopsy forceps or a snare-wire. Repeated examination of patients has demon-strated predictable patterns of recurrence, and histologic studies of the polyps has revised our concept for managing this problem. Research undertaken with organ and tissue culture techniques on the retrieved specimens is stimulating further investigations on the etiology and development and possible growth patterns of carcinomatous tissue.

Several thousand polyps have been removed in our unit with low morbidity and no mortality and, at least to me, colonoscopy seems the procedure of choice for managing polyps.

INSTRUMENTS

Colonoscopes are constantly undergoing change in design, length and visual capabilities. The instruments are expensive and durable and, if improperly handled, may require frequent and expensive repairs.

The basic instrument design is similar for all five major manufacturers of endoscopic equipment in the United States: American Cystoscope Makers, Inc. (ACMI); Fujinon Optical, Inc.; Machida America, Inc.; Olympus Corporation of America; and Pentax Precision Instrument Corporation (Figs. 1-26, Tables 1-5).

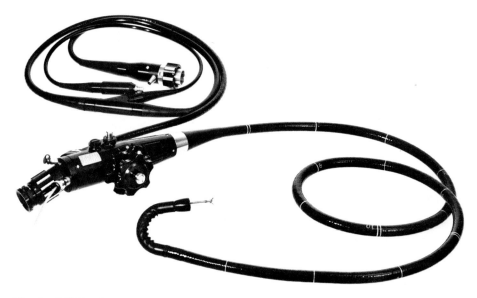

Fig. 1. ACMI colonoscope.

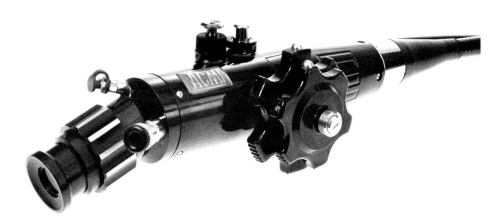

Fig. 2. Control unit of ACMI colonoscope.

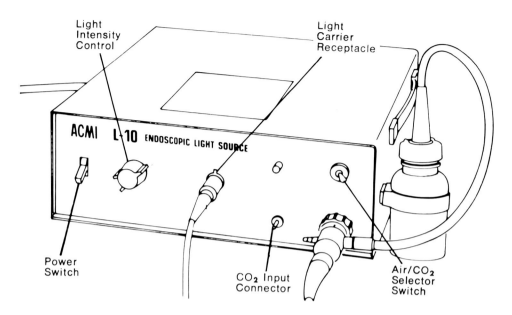

Fig. 3. *ACMI L-10 endoscopic light source.*

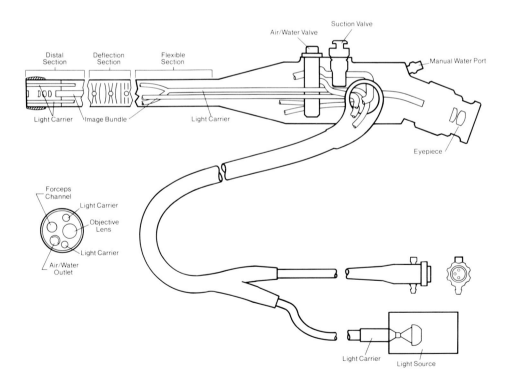

Fig. 4. *Image and illumination systems of ACMI colonoscope.*

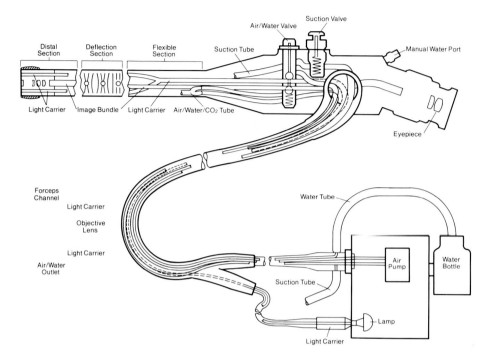

Fig. 5. *Air, irrigation and suction systems of ACMI colonoscope.*

Table 1. ACMI Colonoscopes: Specifications

	TX-91	TX-91R	TX-91S
Working length (mm)	160	110	65
Total length (mm)	187	137	92
Field of view	75°		
Focal depth	2-80 mm		
Adjustable ocular	± 4 diopters		
Diameter of distal end (tip)	13.5 mm		
Diameter of flexible section	13 mm		
Deflection capability	up 180°, down 180°, right 180°, left 180°		
Diameter of forceps channel	3.3 mm		
Air feed, water feed, suction	automatic		

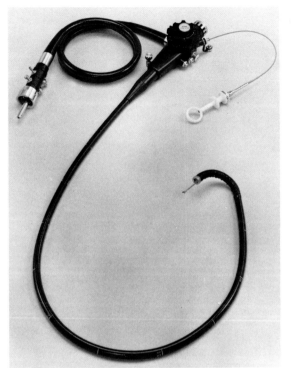

Fig. 6. Fujinon colonoscope.

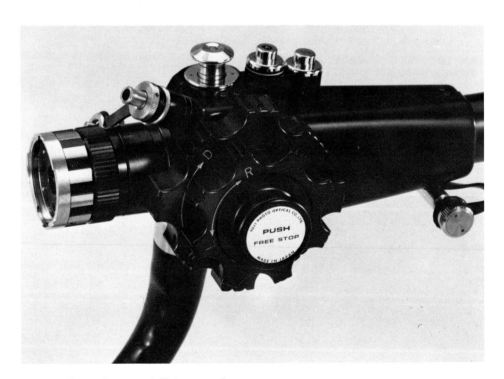

Fig. 7. Control unit of Fujinon colonoscope.

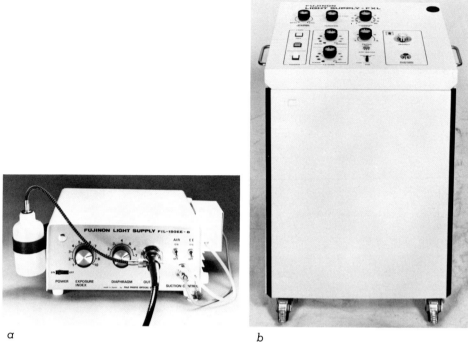

a   b

Figs. 8a and 8b. Fujinon light sources.

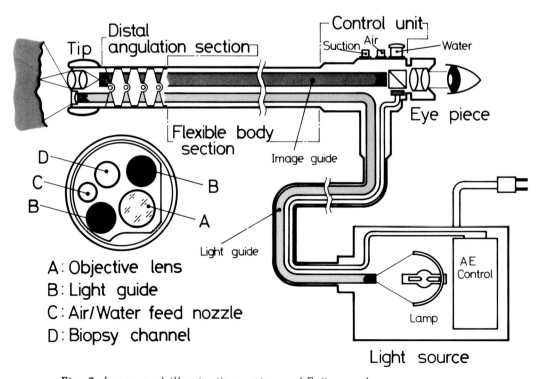

A: Objective lens
B: Light guide
C: Air/Water feed nozzle
D: Biopsy channel

Fig. 9. Image and illumination systems of Fujinon colonoscope.

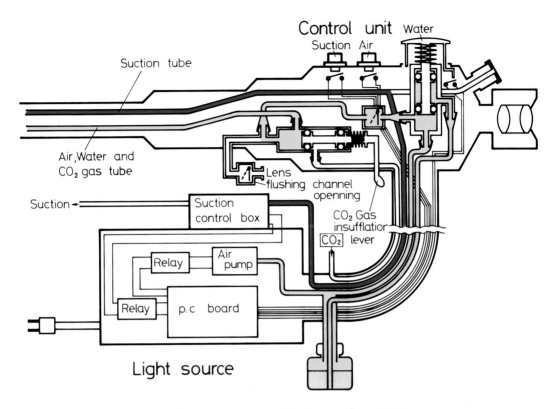

Fig. 10. *Air, irrigation and suction systems of Fujinon colonoscope.*

Table 2. Fujinon Colonoscopes: Specifications

	COLON-M2	COLON-L2	COLON-S2	SG-E
Working length (mm)	1,340	1,835	1,110	725
Total length (mm)	1,500	1,995	1,270	885
Field of view		105°		
Observation range		4-120 mm		
Focus adjustment		fixed		
Diameter of distal end (tip)		13ϕ		
Diameter of flexible section		13ϕ		
Bending capability	up 180°, down 180°, right 160°, left 160°			
Diameter of forceps channel		2.8ϕ		
Air feed, water feed, suction		automatic		

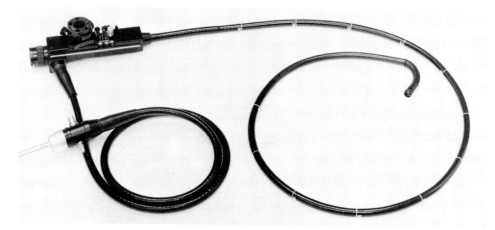

Fig. 11. Machida colonoscope.

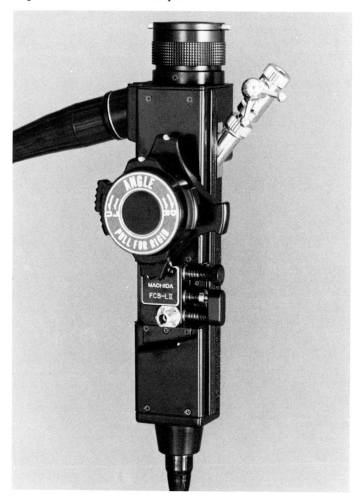

Fig. 12. Control unit of Machida colonoscope.

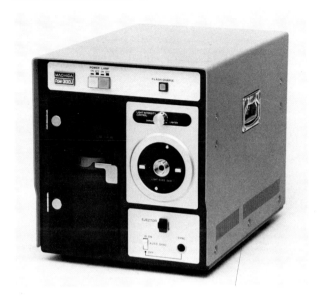

Fig. 13. Machida light source.

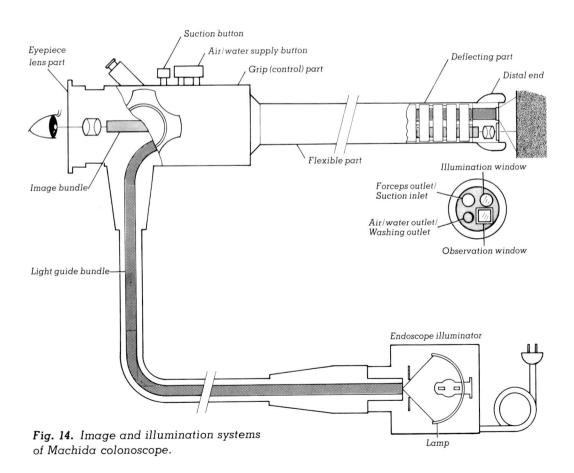

Fig. 14. Image and illumination systems of Machida colonoscope.

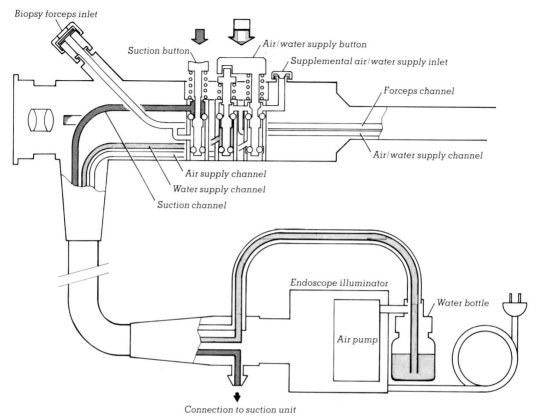

Fig. 15. Air, irrigation and suction systems of Machida colonoscope.

Table 3. Machida Colonoscopes: Specifications

	FCS-MII	FCS-LII	FCS-MWII	FCS-LWII
Total length (mm)	1,266	1,866	1,276	1,876
Working length (mm)	1,060	1,660	1,050	1,650
Apical part				
Diameter (mmϕ)	14.5		16.5	
Length (mm)	8		8	
Flexible part, diameter (mm)	12.7		13.8	
Angle deflection	up 120°, down 120°, right 120°, left 120°			
Angle of vision (forward)	75°		75°	
Depth of focus (fixed) (mm)	5–70		5–70	
Biopsy forceps channel (mmϕ)	2.6		3.8	
Maximum inner diameter (mmϕ)			2.6	

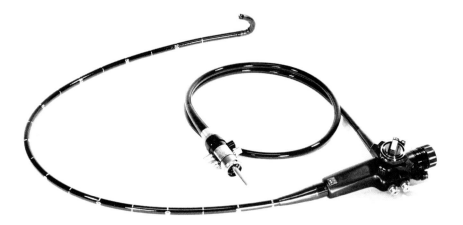

Fig. 16. Olympus colonoscope.

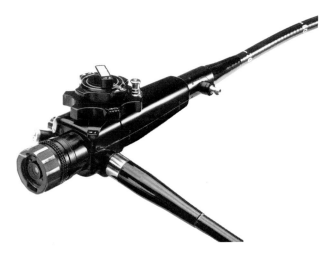

Fig. 17. Control unit of Olympus col-onoscope.

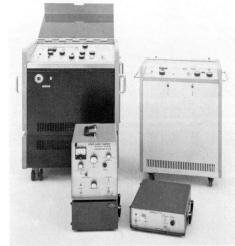

Fig. 18. Olympus light sources.

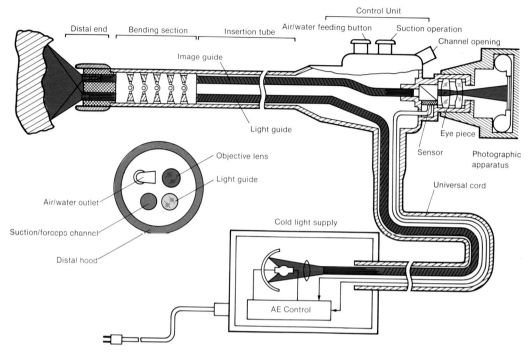

Fig. 19. *Image and illumination systems of Olympus colonoscope.*

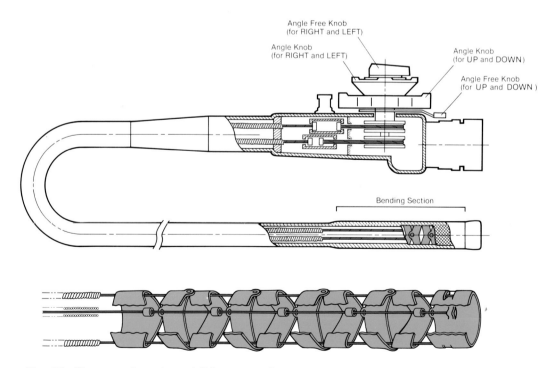

Fig. 20. *Tip control section of Olympus colonoscope.*

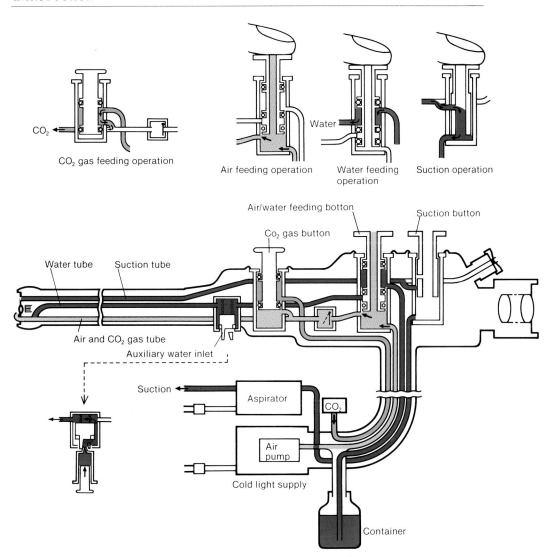

Fig. 21. *Air, irrigation and suction systems of Olympus colonoscope.*

Table 4. Olympus Colonoscopes: Specifications

	CF-MB3R	CF-1B	CF-LB3R	CF-1TS	TCF-1S	TCF-2L2	CF-HM
Optical system							
Angle of view field	85°	85°	85°	90°	85°	85°	70°
Depth of view field (mm)	10-10 (fixed focus)	10-10 (fixed focus)	10-10 (fixed focus)	8-100 (fixed focus)	8-100 (fixed focus)	10-100 (fixed focus)	2.3-100 (adjustable focus)
Distal end							
Outer diameter (mm)	13.6	13.6	13.6	14	16	16.2	14.6
Bending section							
Range of tip bending	180° up, 180° down, 160° right, 160° left	180° up, 180° down, 160° right, 160° left	180° up, 180° down, 160° right, 160° left	180° up, 180° down, 160° right, 160° left	170° up, 170° down, 140° right, 140° left	170° up, 170° down, 140° right, 140° left	180° up, 180° down, 160° right, 160° left
Maximum tip bending	230°	230°	230°	230°	210°	210°	230°
Insertion tube							
Outer diameter (mm)	13.7	13.7	13.7	14.2	16	16.3	14.4
Length							
Working length (mm)	1,035	1,435	1,785	680	680	1,655	1,420
Total length (mm)	1,270	1,670	2,020	915	915	1,900	1,670
Biopsy forceps							
Channel inner diameter (mm)	2.8	2.8	2.8	3.7	5	2.8 (S channel) / 3.7 (L channel)	2.8
Minimum visible distance from distal end (mm)	5	5	5	4	4	5 (S channel) / 6 (L channel)	8
Photography							
Still photography / Cinematography	automatic exposure linked with Olympus Cold Light supply; C-mount adaptors available						

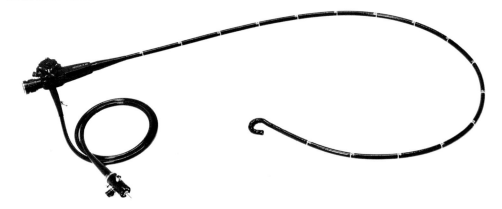

Fig. 22. Pentax colonoscope.

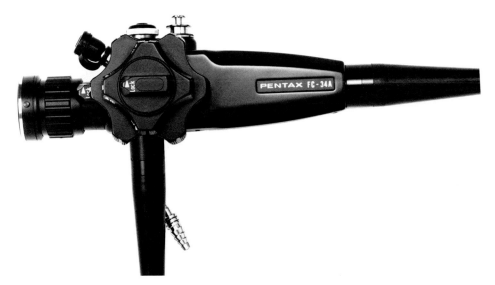

Fig. 23. Control unit of Pentax colonoscope.

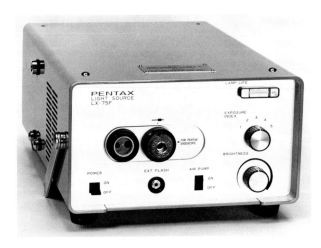

Fig. 24. Pentax light source.

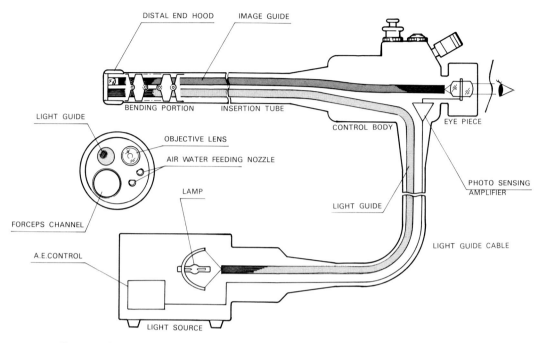

Fig. 25. *Image and illumination systems of Pentax colonoscope.*

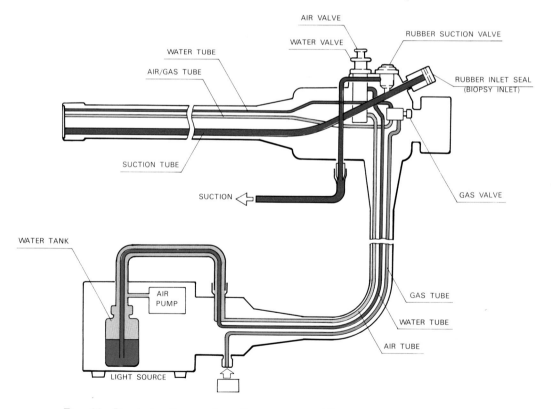

Fig. 26. *Air, irrigation and suction systems of Pentax colonoscope.*

Table 5. Pentax Colonoscopes: Specifications

	FS-34A	FC-34MA	FC-34LA
Angle of viewing field (forward view)		95°	
Depth of viewing field (mm)		3-100	
Diopter		+2 to −8	
Distal rigid portion			
Diameter (mm)		11.5	
Length (mm)		13	
Tip deflection		up 180°, down 180°, right 100°, left 100°	
Insertion tube diameter (mm)		11.5	
Insertion tube working length (mm)	700	1280	1500
Diameter of working channel (mm)		3.5	
Total length (mm)	870	1585	1805

These companies produce high-quality instruments with good service policies. Personal preferences or training determine individual choices of instruments; no substantial advantage of one over another is obvious. Most of our experience has been obtained with the colonoscopes made by Olympus Corporation, although devices by the other four manufacturers have been used as well.

An endoscope contains fine coated glass fibers, as described above, an air channel (through which carbon dioxide may also be insufflated), and a suction and biopsy channel (through which biopsy forceps, snare or brush may be placed). The scopes measure approximately 1.5 cm in diameter and are 105-185 cm long. Because of the flexibility of the fiber bundles, the tip of the instrument may be maneuvered in almost any direction by a dial control on the main body of the scope. The flexibility varies with each manufacturer.

Several types of colonoscopes are available, differentiated by length. They include 105-cm, 130-cm, 160-cm, and 185-cm models and recently a 60-cm model described as a "flexible sigmoidoscope" that may be inserted to the proximal descending colon. This last scope has been the subject of some controversy because it may appeal to many physicians who have no endoscopic training. Its advantages, if any, over partial insertion of a longer instrument are unclear.

The instrument is attached to a light source, which may be a self-standing model or an easily transported table model. The light source generally contains appropriate switches for direct viewing as well as for still photographs, movies and videotapes. The light source usually contains the power source. The colonoscope is also attached to an irrigating fluid reservoir and suction unit. In some manufacturer's models, the fluid reservoir and air insufflator are in the same unit. With an adapter added to the eyepiece, a movie or still photographic camera or video recording device may be used.

ADDRESSES OF ENDOSCOPE MANUFACTURERS

1. American Cystoscope Makers, Inc.
   300 Stillwater Avenue
   Stanford, CT 06902
   (203) 357-8300

2. Fujinon Optical, Inc.
   672 White Plains Road
   Scarsdale, NY 10583
   (914) 472-9802

3. Machida America, Inc.
   65 Oak Street
   Norwood, NJ 07648
   (201) 767-7350

4. Olympus Corporation of America
   4 Nevada Drive
   New Hyde Park, NY 11042
   (516) 488-3880

5. Pentax Precision Instrument Corporation
   55 Oak Street
   Norwood, NJ 07648
   (201) 767-6800

2

Endoscopy Unit

HOSPITAL ENDOSCOPY UNIT

The endoscopy unit should be designed for simple and efficient patient management. The physical design should support this goal by allowing convenience and mobility. The ultimate goal is to have an independently functioning unit for gastrointestinal endoscopy with its own well-trained staff. Obviously, some institutions cannot meet this need, and surgical operating rooms or the x-ray department must be used instead. In other institutions, all endoscopy is carried out in the same unit. These conditions obviously limit physician scheduling and working with specialized personnel.

The endoscopy unit is equipped as follows:

PERSONNEL
· scrub nurse per room
· 1 circulating nurse per room
· 1 endoscopy assistant (e.g., physician, physician's assistant, nurse or training technician)
· 1 nurse's aide for general nursing assistance
· 1 x-ray technician (optional)
· Secretarial pool (one to four secretaries)
· Endoscopy fellow, resident, research assistant or photographer (optional)

SPACE REQUIREMENTS
· Secretarial office
· Waiting room
· Preparation room
· Recovery room

· Examination room
· Fluoroscopy room
· Instrument room (optional)
· Doctor's consultation office
· Dressing room
· Storage room
· Nurse's room
· Bathrooms
· Dictation room

Our patients include ambulatory patients (those who come to our unit for a specific procedure and are discharged after a sufficient recovery period), hospitalized patients and patients transferred from another hospital via ambulance for a specific procedure and then returned to their original institution.

Personnel

Secretaries

Scheduling is done by secretaries. Patients are usually referred by their physicians, who call directly for appointments. The secretaries also obtain a brief summary of the patient's chief complaints, present medications and the availability of x-ray films. We attempt to speak directly with the referring physician. The patient is informed of the routine preparation (if an outpatient) and general procedure. Outpatients are advised to bring a companion to accompany them home after the procedure. Hospitalized patients are scheduled by their private physicians or hospital staff in charge of the case. The secretaries also process patient charts as they enter and leave the unit.

Circulating Nurse

The circulating nurse is responsible for monitoring the patient in the perioperative period. She calls the wards for the inpatients and is thus the liaison with the floor nurse. She thus obtains the other nurses' cooperation and discusses any special postoperative instructions. She is also responsible for transferring patients from the waiting areas to the examination rooms and then to recovery rooms or wards.

Nurse's Aide

The nurse's aide assists with enema preparation, transfer of patients and necessary laundry changes.

Scrub Nurse

The scrub nurse works in the examination room with the physician. She is responsible for drawing up and recording all medications used, checking the instruments, setting them up and cleaning them after each procedure. She also must prepare all polypectomy snares, set up and check the cautery equipment, operate the biopsy forceps and cytology brush and inject contrast material when necessary. Her most important duty is to monitor patients and inform physicians of their patients' condition during the procedure. In addition, any specimens removed are fixed in formalin and labeled for pathologic examination.

Endoscopy Resident or Fellow

The endoscopy resident or fellow has several functions in our unit, aside from learning endoscopic skills. Before the procedure, he or she screens all patients by taking a history and doing a brief physical examination. Once the patient is properly positioned, the resident or fellow administers intravenous medications or begins intravenous lines, as required. He or she assists during the procedure with abdominal manipulation (see page 61) and polypectomy. The resident or fellow is responsible for chart preparation, dictation of procedures and postoperative orders. All hospitalized patients are seen by the resident or fellow after each procedure, at which time they are examined and any questions answered.

X-ray Technician

Our unit has a full-time x-ray technician who is responsible for the care of the x-ray equipment and is available for both taking and processing films.

Research Assistant

A research assistant is usually present during procedures to help collect specimens for ongoing studies and to compile statistics. It may not be practical to have a research assistant in all institutions; I mention this possibility to provide a better idea of the potential of a fully functioning unit.

Layout of Endoscopy Unit

Fig. 27 illustrates our hospital endoscopy unit. It provides maximum mobility for personnel and equipment. The waiting room is separated from the unit. It is

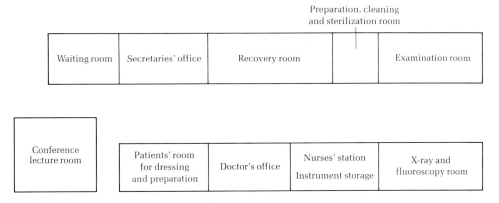

Fig. 27. Layout of a hospital endoscopy unit.

comfortable and allows a place for patients' companions to wait close enough to the unit to transmit information concerning the patient.

The secretaries' office is connected to the waiting room by a small window to facilitate communication.

Across from the secretaries' office is the preparation and patient locker room, where patients remove their clothes and change into examining gowns. Some ambulatory patients cannot properly prepare themselves at home. Such patients are identified at the time of the appointment; they receive enemas in the adjoining bathroom of the preparation room.

Our recovery room has a six-stretcher capacity in addition to chairs for ambulatory patients to use while waiting their turn for the procedure. Curtains separate waiting and recuperating patients. An oxygen tank and emergency cart is nearby and includes an up-to-date emergency drug box, intubation and cut-down set, Ambu bag, and a monitor and electrocardiograph. A telephone to use if a cardiac arrest occurs is located just outside the recovery room.

The physician's office and nurses' locker room directly face the recovery room. Lockers are placed here for personal belongings of the staff. This locale is convenient if the help of other physicians or nurses is needed in the recovery room.

The instrument and supply room is provided for storing endoscopes and ancillary supplies. There is also a sink with appropriate detergents for cleaning equipment.

Two examination rooms occupy the end of the corridor. One room contains the fluoroscopy unit and developer. Both rooms are equipped with individual medication cabinets, holding devices for the endoscopes, sinks, supplies used during the procedure (e.g., gloves and gauze pads) within the cabinets, an area for writing charts and dictating histories and x-ray view boxes. Because our fluoroscopy room is commodious, a special sink for cleansing the instruments is available. All x-ray accessories are kept within the room (lead aprons and gloves), as is additional film. Both rooms contain a standard light source, suction machine, cautery and coagulating unit and an instrument table for immediately needed supplies, such as gloves and lubricating jelly.

The examining room also contains a completely stocked, mobile emergency endoscopy cart checked daily by a unit nurse. This cart contains a portable light source, small suction unit, mouth pieces, local anesthetic, gauze, gloves, biopsy forceps, ancillary teaching attachment and syringes. Intravenous medications are usually obtained from the ward where the patient is located.

We have found that our setup is efficient in handling our workload, which can be quite extensive, and in accommodating a sizable staff of endoscopists. Our patients benefit from our well-organized routine. Our facilities allow us to serve a greater variety of patients safely.

The key to a successful endoscopy unit is to organize it for facile management. To achieve this goal, the personnel within the unit must be able to work with the hospital nursing staff and messenger service. Ambulatory patients must be given clear instructions and feel that the personnel are attentive and available to answer all questions. And, most important, the personnel must be well trained in their particular skills so that the entire unit can function smoothly.

EXAMINING ROOM EQUIPMENT

1. A 6-foot long, flat table with storage space
2. Light source
3. Suction machine
4. Electrosurgical unit
5. Changing area (if inpatient office)
6. Instrument table (for medications, scope, suction and possible cautery device, charts, surgical jelly, gloves and 4 × 4's)
7. Fluoroscopy unit, x-ray unit, lead aprons and gloves

OFFICE ENDOSCOPY

Many endoscopic procedures may be done in a properly equipped private office. The selection of patients for a hospital or office procedure depends on age, general medical condition and diagnosis; whether a patient is already hospitalized also must be taken into account.

Usually, elderly patients (over age 70) with cardiovascular disease, patients with multiple medical problems and those with confirmed polyps are admitted to a hospital or are seen as hospital outpatients. All others may be examined in the office.

The office arrangement is similar to the hospital setup, although on a smaller scale.

The secretarial pool is present, and one or two trained technicians should be available. An endoscopy assistant (physician or nurse) completes the office staff.

The number of examining rooms needed depends on the number of patients examined. We use seven rooms, including one with fluoroscopic capability (Fig. 28).

An examining room should include the following:

1. A 6-foot long, flat table for positioning patients. The table may contain several built-in storage cabinets (Fig. 29).
2. A 4 × 2-foot instrument console designed to make best use of the limited space available (Fig. 30).
3. A long, vertical sidearm with a hook can be built onto the table for suspending the endoscope. The surface of the table is divided into various partitions, including separate sections for medications (diazepam, meperidine, naloxone), lubricating jelly, tissues and gauze, glove box, specimen bottles and occult blood slides.
4. A compartment under the top section of the console is used to house the light source. A larger compartment below this level houses the suction machine and irrigating container.
5. An electrosurgical unit can be kept on a rolling cart for easy transfer from room to room.

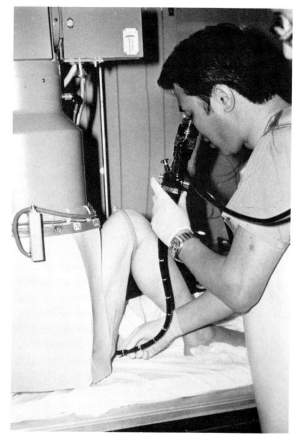

Fig. 28. Colonoscopy being performed under fluoroscopic control. The patient is placed in the supine position with the right knee flexed.

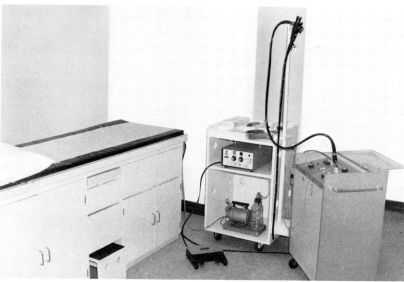

Fig. 29. Endoscopic examination room in the author's office. Homemade examination table, light source, suction cabinet and instrument hanger are shown.

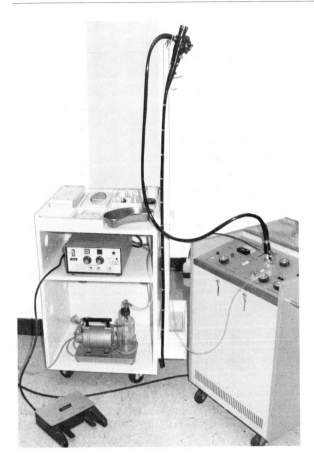

Fig. 30. A homemade instrument cabinet. The scope is hung before and after the examination. Medications, syringes, specimen bottles, paper towels, gloves and tissues are placed in divided compartments.

6. A cubicle or curtain should be provided behind which the patient may comfortably change his or her clothes.

7. A combined instrument room and laboratory is also necessary to house and clean the various scopes. In addition, this area is used to store an autoclave, cleaning agents, microscope, centrifuge and medication cabinets. Resuscitative equipment and an emergency "crash" box for use during respiratory or cardiac arrest are stored here as well. Shelves may be added for general storage of x-ray film, journals, books and photographic equipment.

8. A secretary's office, waiting room and consultation room complete the office layout.

3

Cleaning Colonoscopes and Ancillary Apparatus

There are several reasons why an integral part of colonoscopy is the care and proper cleaning of instruments. First of all, by conscientiously handling and cleaning a colonoscope, the user protects the integrity of the instrument, thus insuring that it will function properly and last a long time. Secondly, care must be taken to protect patients, endoscopy assistants and endoscopists from potentially dangerous transmissable diseases. Thirdly, the operator should consider the instrument an extension of him- or herself and treat it accordingly.

Examination of Instrument

First carefully examine the instrument to look for any damage to its external surface. Cleaning agents may harm the delicate internal mechanism if breaks in surface integrity are present. Things to look for are cracks in the skin of the shaft, water under the optical objective and poor functioning of air or suction channels. Do not immerse an instrument if any such condition exists. Send it immediately for repair.

Mechanical Cleaning

Clean the instrument immediately after the operative procedure to prevent crusting of solid matter on its external surface. In addition, gross contamination from fecal material is avoided. It has also been reported that evaporation leads to the formation of corrosive salts, which may damage the scope.

After the procedure and while the scope is still attached to the light source and suction machine, first submerge the tip of the scope into a container with a 30%-40% alcohol solution. Place a finger on the suction button of the instrument, then suction alcohol until a clear return is obtained. Detach the cord of the water container leading to the instrument. Then, place a fingertip against the opening at the base of the cord. With the other hand, push the air insufflation button until all water is cleared from the scope. Next, detach the instrument from the light source and suction machine, and take it to the utility room for mechanical cleaning.

It is important to note that the control section and light guide connector must not be immersed in any cleaning solution or allowed to get wet.

The next step is the mechanical cleaning of the scope. Suspend the instrument from an appropriate hook. Wash down the insertion tube with any nonabrasive surgical soap diluted with lukewarm water (20% soap, 80% water); use short stroking motions. Then, rinse the insertion tube with water. Next, remove the tip, then clean, rinse and replace it. Next, wash down the insertion tube with a 70% alcohol solution. Then, rinse the biopsy channel with water, and run through a wire brush to remove any particulate matter. Blow dry the channel with a rubber bulb and hang it to drain. If it is to be used immediately, dry it mechanically with soft toweling.

Disinfection and Sterilization

A thorough cleaning is required before the insertion tube is disinfected or the fiberscope is sterilized. Disinfection is necessary to remove any pathogenic organisms. Most manufacturers recommend using a solution of iodophor (Betadine) or glutaraldehyde (Cidex). When used properly, these solutions do not damage the fiberscope.

First, wipe the insertion tube with a disinfectant. Then, suck the solution through the channel after immersing the instrument tip. Soak the insertion tube in the solution for 20 minutes or less. Do not oversoak the tube or soak the control section for fear of damage. Remove the disinfectant by washing and suctioning with tap water. Then, wash the instrument again and suction with 70% alcohol; hang the instrument to dry.

Sterilization of the colonoscope is necessary in:

1. Cases of infectious hepatitis
2. Cases of infectious bowel disease (e.g., amebiasis, shigella or salmonella, etc.)
3. As a reverse precaution in immunologically depressed patients.

Sterilization with ethylene oxide gas can be done without damage, provided that the fiberscope is clean and the following conditions are met:

1. Temperature is less than 57°C (135°F)
2. Pressure is less than 20 psi
3. Aeration time is about 24 hours at room temperature or 12 hours at 50°C (122°F) in an aeration chamber

The biopsy valve, distal hood or suction adapter should be removed and sterilized separately.

Cleaning Accessories

Snare-wire
To clean the snare-wire, first remove it from the polyethylene sheath. Clean both the wire and sheath with surgical soap and water. Run alcohol through the tubing. Then blow dry with a syringe. Thread the wire back into the polyethylene tubing. Last, sterilize the device with ethylene oxide.

Biopsy Forceps
First wash the forceps with surgical soap, then rinse it well with water. (Sometimes it is necessary to soak the forceps in peroxide to remove any clotted blood.) Then sterilize the forceps with ethylene oxide.

4

Endoscopy Record

A record of the patient's endoscopy examination should be brief and concise because of space limitations. However, it should contain several key entries (Fig. 31) including medication record, pertinent medical history and procedure performed and type of instrument used.

The medication record is a helpful aid in repeat colonoscopies. If the patient had any discomfort at an earlier examination or perhaps was slightly over-medicated, a notation in the medication record would indicate how to alter the dose.

A brief pertinent medical history should be obtained and recorded on a checkoff list. This list should include the following: rectal bleeding; change in bowel habit and its duration; and abdominal pain and its location.

Also, significant medical and surgical diseases should be ascertained, as should dates of any surgical intervention.

Present medications are of importance as well.

The family history should include questions regarding cancer (especially of the colon and rectum), colonic polyps, inflammatory bowel disease and other conditions.

The procedure should be recorded (e.g., colonoscopy-polypectomy or biopsy), as should the instrument used. Also, if a splinting device or fluoroscopy was needed, it should be recorded as well. It is also important to indicate the level to which the scope was inserted. This information should include the anatomic location and the distance in centimeters from the anal verge (e.g., cecum, 115 cm). There are several points to consider.

It is difficult to give an exact length with regard to distance of insertion, especially beyond the sigmoid. However, a reasonable estimate can be indicated. With the 105-cm instrument that we usually use, with the colon straightened, we find the following distances:

· Rectosigmoid, 12-15 cm
· Midsigmoid, 25-30 cm
· Proximal sigmoid, 30-40 cm
· Mid-descending colon, 30-50 cm
· Splenic flexure, 40-70 cm

ENDOSCOPIC REPORT

LOWER GI EXAMINATION

NAME	AGE	SEX	DICTATED

ADDRESS | TELEPHONE NO.

HOME: | OFFICE:

REFERRED BY: DR. | PRE OPERATIVE DIAGNOSIS | INDICATIONS

TEL NO.:

MEDICATION: | B/P: | PULSE:

TIME: DEMEROL (MG.) VALIUM (MG.) NARCAN (MG.)

SYMPTOMS:

☐ RECTAL BLEEDING ☐ ABDOMINAL PAIN
☐ CHANGE OF BOWEL HABIT ☐ ASYMPTOMATIC
☐ DIARRHEA ☐ OTHER:
☐ CONSTIPATION

PAST HX: ☐ HEART CONDITION
☐ ANTICOAGULANT
☐ HYPERTENSION
☐ HYSTERECTOMY OR PELVIC SURGERY
☐ COLON RESECTION
☐ RECTAL OR COLON POLYP
☐ OTHER

BA ENEMA: ☐ POS. ☐ NEG. ☐ UNCERTAIN

☐ BIOPSY

☐ POLYPECTOMY – NO. OF POLYPS REMOVED

FAMILY HX: ☐ CA.
☐ POLYP
☐ INFLAMMATORY BOWEL DISEASE
☐ OTHER

LEVEL OF INSERTION: UP TO COLON CM.

COLONOSCOPE ( ) MODEL ☐ FLUROSCOPY ☐ SPLINTING DEVICE

SIZE OF LESIONS: CF: 1. 2. 3. 4. 5.

LEVEL: (CM.)

FINDINGS:

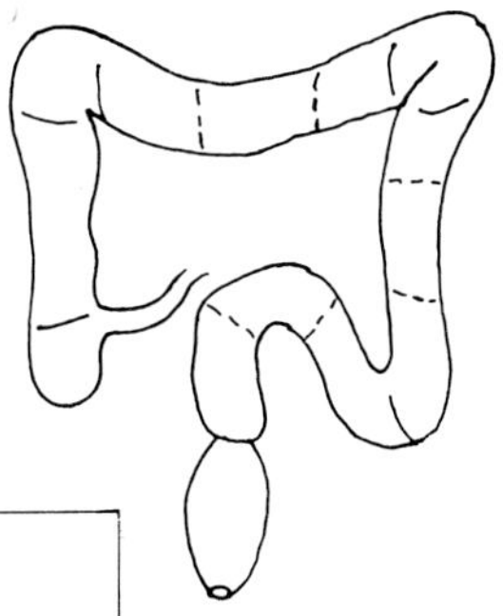

FOLLOW–UP DATES: _____ MONTHS: INPT. OUTPT. OFFICE

DICTATED ☐ YES ☐ NO

ENDOSCOPIC DIAGNOSIS:

SNOP #

_____ _____ MD _____ RN

DATE OF PROCEDURE:

CHART COPY

Fig. 31.

· Midtransverse colon, 50-90 cm
· Hepatic flexure, 70-105 cm
· Cecum, 75-130 cm

Naturally, with bowing of the instrument in a redundant colon or when various colonic loops are present, more scope is inserted than corresponds to actual distance. It is only when the colon has been straightened that a reasonable estimation can be made. An aid that we frequently use relates the distance to the cecum with the ease or difficulty of insertion. That is, a relatively easy insertion to the cecum would be indicated by a distance of 100-115 cm, moderate difficulty by 120 cm and extreme difficulty by 130 cm.

The nature of any pathologic lesions should be accurately described; the size, number, anatomic location and distance from the anal verge in centimeters should be noted. In addition, with regard to polypoid lesions, the following features should be mentioned:

1. Gross description (e.g., smooth, lobulated, villous appearing or ulcerated)
2. Pedunculated or sessile, narrow base or wide base (if pedunculated, describe the stalk as being short, heavy, long, etc.)
3. Size
4. Number
5. Distribution

Again, with regard to level, the exact distance may be difficult to determine because of the above-mentioned problems. However, using the rough distances cited above, or taking the average between the distance of the lesion from the anal verge during insertion and the distance during withdrawal, may help pinpoint the abnormality.

If one wishes to more accurately pinpoint a lesion that has been documented by barium enema, fluoroscopic examination can confirm the entry of the scope to the desired level.

It is also helpful to have a diagram of the colon or the endoscopy record sheet, so that the operator can diagrammatically record the nature and level of a lesion. This is useful for repeat colonoscopy examinations. In this way, the desired area of reexamination is quickly perused.

5

Indications
and Contraindications

Colonoscopy is an excellent method for evaluating colonic disease, and all patients being scheduled for barium enema studies should be considered for a colonoscopy.

INDICATIONS

Our indications for colonoscopy are as follows:

1. *Diagnosis.* In the presence of symptoms when x-ray studies are negative or equivocal, for confirmation when they are positive and when searching for a source of occult bleeding
2. *Biopsy.* Either to confirm the presence of a malignant lesion with tissue sections or to establish the nature of the disease when inflammatory in origin and/or when associated malignant degeneration is present
3. *Polyps.* For therapeutic removal, to search for additional polyps or associated carcinoma when the polyp has been demonstrated and to search for polyps in the presence of known carcinoma
4. *Follow-up.* After bowel resection for cancer as a means of detecting local recurrence or metachronous lesions, after polypectomy and to evaluate the effectiveness of therapy for inflammatory diseases
5. *Foreign bodies.* Including detection and removal
6. *Screening purposes.* Particularly in early carcinoma detection
7. *Clinical research studies*

CONTRAINDICATIONS

The following conditions should be considered as contraindications for its use:

1. Acute fulminating inflammatory bowel disease
2. Acute diverticulitis with systemic reaction
3. Suspected perforation of the bowel
4. Abdominal and iliac aneurysm
5. Paralytic ileus with peritonitis
6. Partial or complete intestinal obstruction
7. Acute inflammatory disease of the anus

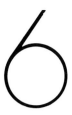

Preparation
and Medications

A well-cleansed bowel is required for a proper and safe colonoscopic examination and electrosurgery. Traditional preparation of the bowel requires dietary restriction, laxatives and enemas. The details of bowel preparation for both colonoscopy and colonoscopic polypectomy may vary somewhat, but all have the same aim: to obtain an adequately cleansed bowel.

BOWEL PREPARATION

Routine Preparation

Our standard preparation of the colon is as follows:

1. Clear fluids for 24 hours before the procedure
2. Ten ounces of citrate of magnesia or 45-60 ml of castor oil in the late afternoon of the day prior to examination
3. A warm tap water enema until a clear return is obtained (usually up to two quarts) 2 hours before the procedure

Unsatisfactory bowel preparation is unusual with this regimen.

Preparation for Inflammatory Bowel Disease and Diarrheal Disorders

Preparation regimens should be adjusted if inflammatory bowel disease and/or diarrheal disorders exist. Patients are usually prepared by requesting them to take clear liquids for 24-36 hours and warm tap water enemas, until clear, the evening before the procedure and the morning of the examination. A cathartic is either given in small doses or omitted.

Preparation for Constipation or Advanced Diverticular Disease

If the patient is known to have chronic constipation or advanced diverticular disease of the colon, more vigorous preparation may be required. Patients may require clear liquids and oral purgatives for two days.

Preparation for Colonic Stricture or Obstruction

Patients with partial or total colonic obstruction should receive nothing by mouth. They are given frequent tap water enemas or high colonic irrigations. If, during the examination, the patient has been found to be unsatisfactorily cleansed, 500-1500 ml of tap water or normal saline should be introduced through the biopsy channel of the instrument and the scope withdrawn. After the fecal material has been expelled in the next 2-3 hours, colonoscopy can be attempted again. No cathartics should be given to such patients.

Preparation for Young Children

Bowel preparation for a young child is usually 5-10 ounces of citrate of magnesia or 0.5-1.5 oz of castor oil the evening before the procedure and one tap water enema 2 hours before endoscopy. The cleansing regimen should be determined on the basis of age, weight and general condition of the patient.

Saline Irrigation Method

This method is gaining popularity among colonoscopists. The advantages of this preparation are:

1. Rapidity (usually requires 3-4 hours)
2. Well tolerated by patients
3. Enemas unnecessary
4. Inexpensive
5. Causes no histologic changes in the mucosa

Saline solution (3,000-4,000 ml) can be given to patients either by mouth or via nasogastric tube.
  The saline lavage method is as follows:

1. Clear fluids for 12 hours
2. 1,000 ml. of saline given, over a period of 1 hour, 6 hours before the procedure
3. A second liter of saline given, over the next hour, 5 hours before the examination
4. A third liter of saline given, over the next hour, 4 hours before the examination
5. A fourth liter of saline given, over the next hour, 3 hours before the examination.

The patient should stop drinking the saline solution when evacuation per rectum becomes clear or when 4,000 ml of saline intake is completed. Oral saline lavage preparation may be carried out in the office, hospital or even at home. It is not advised for patients with cardiac disease, those taking steroids or those with hypertension or renal disease, in whom salt retention may be unsafe.

Mannitol Preparation

Mannitol preparation is a more recent addition to the above-described methods. One liter of 10% mannitol is used for preparation and is given by mouth 5 hours before the examination.

1. Patients should be kept on clear fluids for 24 hours.
2. 100 ml. of mannitol should be given on two occasions, 30 minutes apart.
3. 200 ml. of mannitol should be repeated every 30 minutes four times.

It is wise to monitor the patient's blood pressure, pulse and weight. This preparation is not advised if polypectomy is planned since bowel explosions have been reported with mannitol.

MEDICATIONS

Medication regimens before and during the procedure vary to some degree. Each endoscopist should establish a program to provide comfort and safety during the colonoscopic procedure. Not all colonoscopists provide premedication, particularly for outpatients and the elderly. Depending on the needs or the attitude of the patient, the following medications can be used:

Meperidine (Demerol), diazepam (Valium), pentazocine (Talwin), nalbuphine (Nubain), sodium phenobarbital or phenergan administered either intramuscularly or intravenously. We usually administer meperidine (25-75 mg) and/or diazepam (2.5-10 mg) intravenously. Glucagon (1.0 mg) intravenously or Dicyclomine (Bentyl) (10 mgm-20 mgm) intramuscularly is used occasionally as an antispasmotic agent.

The use of anticholinergics has largely been eliminated because these drugs frequently produce marked distention and abdominal cramps and may be associated with prolonged retention of air inflated during the course of the examination.

The use of general anesthesia is not recommended. However, medication regimens should be adjusted according to the specific psychologic needs and general medical condition of the patient.

7

Colonoscopy and X-ray Examination

COLONOSCOPY AND BARIUM ENEMA

These two modalities serve to complement one another in diagnosing colon pathology. Although newer methods of fine air-contrast studies are being added to the radiologist's armamentarium, some lesions can still be missed. Colonoscopy enables physicians to accurately localize and biopsy the lesion. It is also useful in discovering lesions not seen on x-ray examination. A well-prepared patient and an exacting radiologist may almost duplicate an endoscopist's findings. Certainly the diagnostic accuracy is enhanced with the combination of these procedures.

The usual diagnostic workup for suspected colonic disease includes barium enema, followed by colonoscopy. Many radiologists and gastroenterologists are well trained in the performance of the barium enema, and it is thus easy to obtain. Although increasing, the number of well-trained colonoscopists is still small. Furthermore, an x-ray study provides a helpful map for endoscopists, especially when there are redundant loops of bowel or many diverticula.

In a recently published prospective study, endoscopy was found to be more accurate than barium enema, especially for diagnosing small polyps and carcinomas, but the procedures were considered complementary. In this series, 30% of the patients had incomplete colonoscopies; that is, the endoscopist failed to reach the cecum. Our experience is biased by the uneven quality of x-ray films we receive from patients referred from outside our institution.

We have found abnormalities that correlate with symptoms in a great many patients with "negative" x-ray studies. Therefore, our bias is that every patient with suggestive symptoms, particularly rectal bleeding and anemia, should undergo colonoscopy, even if they have a negative barium enema.

USE OF FLUOROSCOPY

Fluoroscopy is used under certain conditions, including the following:

1. To confirm either cecal entry or entry into areas of a suspected lesion as suggested on barium enema
2. For a long, redundant and tortuous sigmoid colon
3. For a sigmoid colon that is sharply angulated or fixed because of a previous surgical procedure or inflammatory disease
4. To demonstrate fistulous tracts with the use of contrast material injected through the colonoscope
5. For use of the splinting device (see page 69)

Increased radiation is harmful to patients, endoscopists, and ancillary personnel, and it can damage the fibers causing a yellowish discoloration.

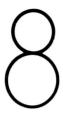

Endoscopic Anatomy
of the Colon

Endoscopists must be aware of the normal anatomy of the colon and its relations to adjacent organs and vessels. An endoscopic view of the colon is quite different from the appearance noted during a surgical procedure or roentgenologic studies. The purpose of this chapter is to familiarize fledgling endoscopists with the normal anatomy of the various segments of the colon and to clearly define landmarks that can be used to recognize the observed segment.

Endoscopists must be able to equate areas seen on barium enema films to the corresponding segments of colon seen through the colonoscope. They must be able to properly identify the cecum, without fluoroscopic assistance, since this tool may not always be available.

The following description of the colon will begin in the anal canal (as do most colonoscopies) and advance proximally.

Anal Canal

The anal canal, while only 3 cm long, must not be ignored in routine endoscopy. The increasing reliance on fiberoptic endoscopy and radiologic examination has unfortunately caused many physicians to omit basic procedures, namely, rectal examination and proctoscopy. We have examined many patients referred with missed and obvious anal abnormalities, including melanoma and squamous carcinoma.

The anal canal begins as a cutaneous canal, changing to a mucosal canal at the dentate line. The color of the mucosa is pale above the dentate line, becoming pink approximately 1.5 cm proximal as the rectum is entered. Careful examination of the anus is made for lesions and internal hemorrhoids.

Rectum

The common belief that the rectum is poorly visualized by the fiberoptic colonoscope is a misconception that must be permanently laid to rest. With proper technique and preparation, the colonoscope is superior to rigid proctosigmoidoscopy to visualize this area.

The rectum extends from the anal canal to the rectosigmoid junction, a distance of approximately 12-15 cm. The portion of the rectum below the pelvic peritoneum is dilated and referred to as the ampulla. Despite its short length, several curves, or angulations, may be present (Fig. 32).

Above the ampulla, the first of the three valves of Houston is seen on the left. The second valve, located on the right, corresponds to the peritoneal reflection. The third valve is also positioned on the left and represents the terminal boundary of the rectum. The area immediately behind each valve must be visualized to avoid missing lesions.

Beginner endoscopists may have trouble recognizing the valves of Houston. They will not, however, have difficulty recognizing the rectosigmoid junction. At this point, the lumen of the rectum no longer continues in its cephalad course but turns downward into the pelvis as it becomes the sigmoid colon.

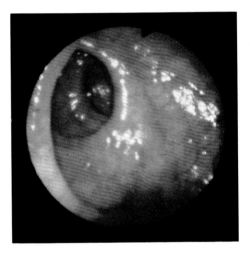 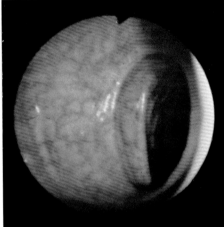

Fig. 32. Endoscopic view of a portion of the rectosigmoid and distal sigmoid colon.   *Fig. 33. Semilunar mucosal folds of the midsigmoid colon.*

Sigmoid Colon

The sigmoid colon (Fig. 33) varies in length from approximately 30 to 60 cm, with an average of 30-40 cm. It is readily recognized by its tubular appearance and by its prominent semilunar haustrae. The lumen usually has a smaller diameter than does the rectum. However, every patient is different, and there is no uniform feature of the haustrae that enables endoscopists to definitively identify the sigmoid colon all the time. They may be forced to rely on knowledge of anatomic landmarks of the rectum and descending colon to determine the boundaries of the sigmoid colon. Pathologic conditions, such as diverticular disease, inflammatory bowel disease and adhesions from previous surgical procedure, can produce angulation, shortening or varying diameters of the lumen.

Descending Colon

The descending colon (Fig. 34) is usually recognized by the sigh of relief from the endoscopist. This reaction occurs because of the anatomic nature of the descending colon, which is composed of about 20-30 cm of tubular colon, fixed on the left colic gutter. This portion of the colon may be easily traversed by the tip of the endoscope in the true neutral position. It is somewhat narrower than the sigmoid and mostly round in shape and appearance. Tension by other structures on the taenia occasionally alters its shape from perfectly round, although it is not triangular, as is the transverse colon.

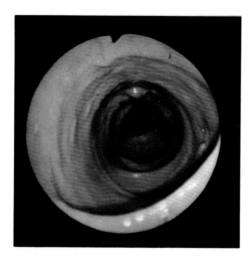

Fig. 34. Tubular view of the descending colon. Folds are less prominent than in the sigmoid or transverse colon. A small polyp is also in view.

Splenic Flexure

The splenic flexure (Fig. 35) marks the end of the easy passage through the descending colon. It often has the appearance of a pouch, because the lumen into the transverse colon is often situated 180 degrees from the axis of the endoscope. Occasionally, the spleen may be seen as a light blue transparency through the colonic wall.

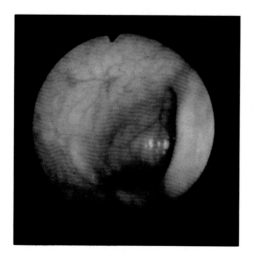

Fig. 35. A view of the splenic flexure as a pouch and mucosal fold.

Transverse Colon

The transverse colon is approximately 45 cm in length. The haustrae have a classic triangular appearance (Figs. 36-38), caused by their three taenial bands. The left transverse colon can be identified by noting and feeling the transmitted pulsation of the aorta. The proximal transverse colon is characterized by the sharp blue-brown liver shadow seen through the colonic wall. This finding indicates that the hepatic flexure has been reached.

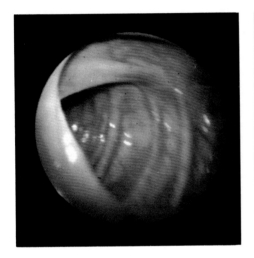

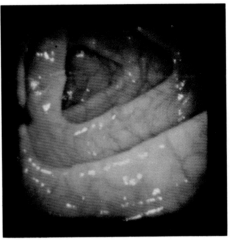

Fig. 36. Left transverse colon. The triangular folds are less prominent than those in the right transverse colon.

Fig. 37. The midtransverse colon with typical triangular folds.

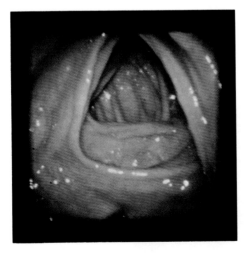

Fig. 38. View of the hepatic flexure.

Hepatic Flexure

The hepatic flexure (Figs. 39 and 40) represents the junction of the horizontal transverse colon and the vertical ascending colon. Due to the relation of the right lobe of the liver to the right transverse colon, the hepatic flexure is usually situated at a 90-degree angle rather than a 180-degree angle, as is the splenic flexure. Once the liver shadow is noted and the hepatic flexure is reached, entrance into the ascending colon is downward and to the right.

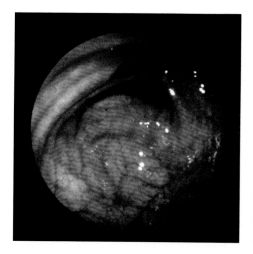

Fig. 39. Hepatic flexure in another patient.

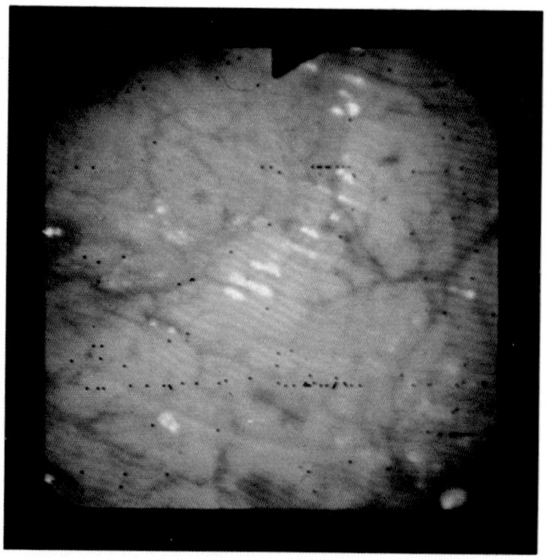

Fig. 40. Hepatic flexure with prominent, bluish liver shadow.

Ascending Colon

The ascending colon (Fig. 41) is about 15 cm long and has many distinguishing features. The diameter of the ascending colon is larger than that of the transverse colon, and it is shaped like a rounded triangle. Approximately 50% of the luminal surface area is encircled by folds rather than the entire circumference. The colonic wall in the ascending colon is usually covered with golden yellow fecal fluid.

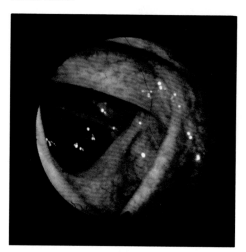

Fig. 41. Typical endoscopic view of the ascending colon. Triangular folds are not contiguous.

Cecum

The cecum (Figs. 42-45) is the portion of the right colon that lies caudad to the ileocecal valve. All three taenia coli converge at the apex of the cecum, usually with the appendiceal orifice at the point of convergence. The ileocecal valve is seen as a prominence along the medial wall. A slight indentation, or concavity, is noted; this feature represents the entrance of the valve. The ileocecal valve can be entered as described in Chapter 9 and the terminal ileum visualized. Lastly, gentle tapping in the right lower quadrant of the abdomen may be seen as an indentation in the cecal contour.

With knowledge of simple anatomy and a few endoscopic "pearls," trained endoscopists should have no difficulty in ascertaining their location inside the colon and thus insure a complete examination.

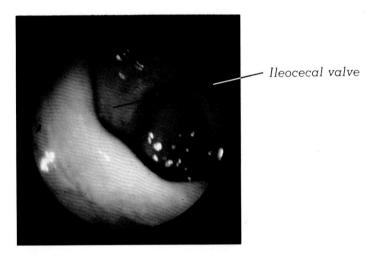

Ileocecal valve

Fig. 42. Side view of the ileocecal valve (type I) and a portion of the cecum.

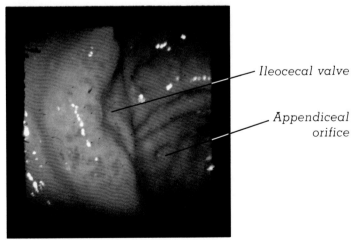

Ileocecal valve

Appendiceal orifice

Fig. 43. Another view of the ileocecal valve; more prominent type (type II). A part of the cecum, including the appendiceal orifice, is also shown.

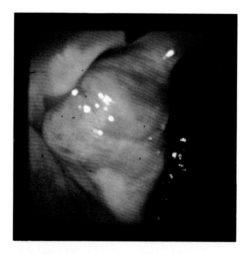

Fig. 44. *Most prominent ileocecal valve (type III), side view, probably associated with lipomatous component.*

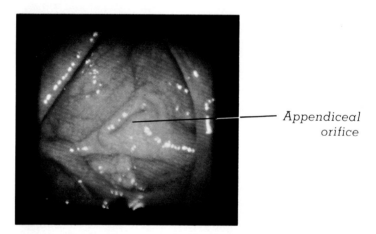

Appendiceal
orifice

Fig. 45. *View of the cecum shows the appendiceal orifice in the center.*

Terminal Ileum

The terminal ileum noted just inside the ileocecal valve has a granular, velvety mucosal lining representing areas of lymphoid hyperplasia. This is more prominent in young persons. Since there are no taenia, the lumen is small and round. The mucosa is generally pinker than colonic mucosa, and the submucosal capillaries are much less prominent (Fig. 46). An inverted appendeceal stump and site of anastomosis can be identified without difficulty (Figs. 47-49).

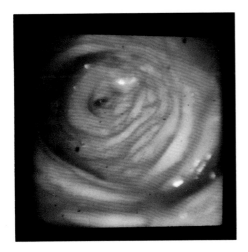 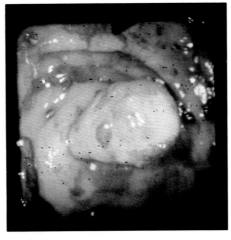

Fig. 46. End-on view of the terminal ileum.

Fig. 47. Inverted appendiceal stump.

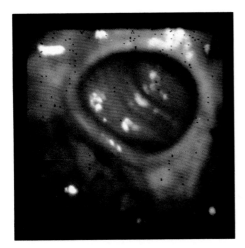 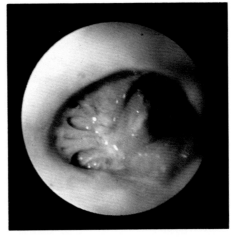

Fig. 48. Ileocolic anastomosis.

Fig. 49. Site of colonic anastomosis shows marked scarring and narrowing with pseudodiverticular orifices, suggesting a technically poor anastomosis.

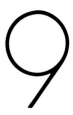

Insertion Techniques

Although colonoscopy has become popular and its application widespread, the proper technique of insertion and advancement of the scope is often not stressed during training. Many experienced endoscopists continue to advance the scope despite patient discomfort and thus require longer instruments to reach the cecum.

A firm understanding of colonic anatomy, torque forces and maneuvers that straighten and shorten the colon are required. To achieve this skill, the operator must learn to handle the instrument by him- or herself during the entire procedure.

As shown in Fig. 50a, the left hand must grasp the control unit of the scope; the control unit is firmly held with the left fourth and fifth fingers and a light touch of the third finger. The index finger is used to push the water air insufflation button and the aspiration button. The left thumb is used only to flex the directional knobs on the control unit.

The right hand should be used only to manipulate the body of the scope. The right hand may also be used to insert the biopsy forceps, the snare-wire and other biopsy channel devices.

The body of the scope is held by the thumb, index finger and middle finger of the right hand for insertion, torque and withdrawal of the instrument.

The most important factors in becoming adept at colonoscopy are:

1. To develop "coordination" between the left thumb motion (flexion of the tip of the instrument) and right hand movement (insertion, withdrawal and torque).
2. To develop a "feel" for the colon by the left thumb and the right hand (a sense of stretching and looping of the colon and straightening of the scope, which prevents perforation).
3. To develop a "timing" of motions between the left index finger (aspiration of air from the colon), the left thumb and the right hand.

The only way to acquire such skill is through repeated examinations of numerous patients. However, I believe one should emphasize the above aspects to avoid poor colonoscopic habits. As with many other technical procedures, proper form is the best way to achieve a masterful and safe technique.

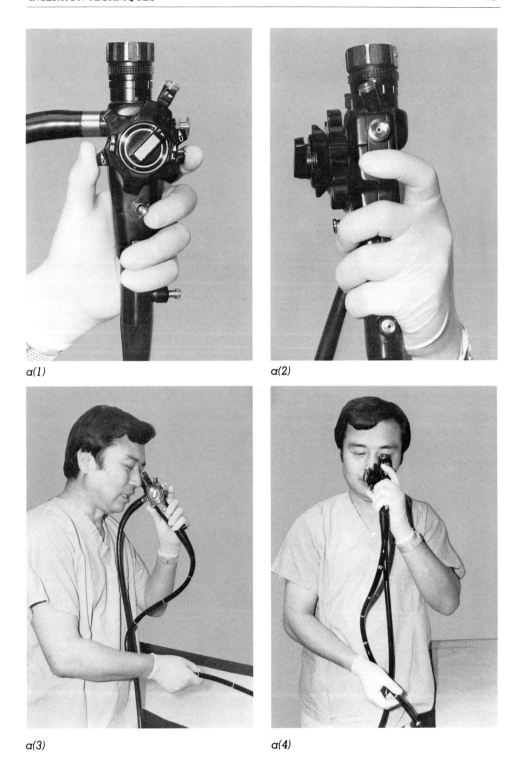

α(1)   α(2)

α(3)   α(4)

Figs. 50α(1–4). *Demonstration of the proper hand grip of the control unit and instrument.*

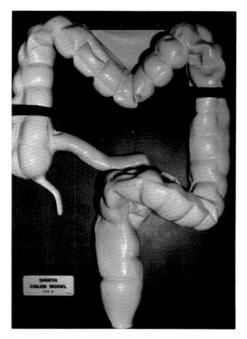

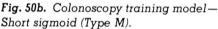

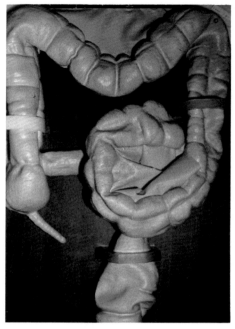

Fig. 50b. *Colonoscopy training model—Short sigmoid (Type M).*

Fig. 50c. *Colonoscopy training model—Long sigmoid (Type L).*

The ability to successfully perform endoscopic procedures with expertise and minimal patient discomfort depends largely upon the technical skill and deftness of the operator. In order to attain these skills, there is, of course, no substitute for actual "hands on" patient experience. However, the finesse required to perform many of the maneuvers necessary in colonoscopy can only be achieved by repetitive training. We have designed and constructed several latex colon models specifically for this purpose (Fig. 50b). In teaching seminars the coordination motions between the control knob and the shaft of the instrument can be practiced under supervision. The insertion, withdrawal, and torque motions are demonstrated on the models and then repetitively carried out by the students. There are basically two ways that the scope may be inserted: either by advancing the scope as one sees the lumen or, in more experienced hands, by torque and withdrawal maneuvers before the lumen comes into view. It is essential that if one inserts the scope and meets resistance, the scope should be withdrawn, simultaneously aspirating air from the lumen. One should not torque the scope when meeting resistance or during insertion. Torquing the scope should only occur during withdrawal of the instrument. These principles are of the utmost importance and should be strongly adhered to during the performance of colonoscopy.

In addition, techniques for colonoscopic polypectomy can be practiced using these models. We have designed several models which represent colon types of varying difficulty (Fig. 50c). These models allow one to practice the alpha maneuver, right turn shortening technique, insertion of the splinting device and other colonoscopic techniques.

In our unit, the patient is placed on the examination table in the left lateral recumbent position. The procedure is started and completed in this position. Intravenous medications are administered to relax both the patient and his or her colon. These medications (e.g., meperidine, diazepam or glucagon) are short acting (approximately 15-20 minutes), and it thus becomes incumbent on the endoscopist to proceed as rapidly as possible. If the patient becomes extremely uncomfortable after 20 minutes, and it is determined that the cause of the discomfort is not excessive stretching of the bowel or perforation but the procedure itself, the endoscopist may administer an additional small dose of medication. At the end of the procedure, we routinely give naloxone intravenously or intramuscularly to counteract the effect of meperidine and allow ambulatory patients to leave the unit with or without a companion after a brief period of rest and observation (about 15-45 minutes).

Examination of the colonoscope reveals several points that will be referred to in the following discussion. Most instruments have the same basic design.

The control head of the endoscope is held comfortably in the left hand with the left thumb applied lightly to the up/down control knob and with the left index finger placed opposite the air channel superiorly enough so that the suction button can also be easily reached with lateral motion of the finger. The third and fourth fingers grasp the base of the head piece in a firm but easy grip, so that the forearm does not easily fatigue and the endoscope will not slip through the operator's fingers. The distal portion of the endoscope is grasped lightly by the right hand. When more directional turn is required, the right/left control on the head of the instrument may be turned with the left thumb, without releasing the distal end of the endoscope with the right hand. This method gives the endoscopist complete control over the tip of the endoscope.

When flexion is mentioned, it refers to motion of the left thumb on the up/down control knob. Flexing this control (or pulling the thumb and wheel in a downward direction) results in flexion of the instrument tip in an upward direction, and extension of the dial causes a downward deflection. If the right hand is used to control the clockwise and counterclockwise rotations and the left thumb is used to control up and down movements of the tip, all directions can be obtained with the endoscopist in complete control of the endoscope.

The objective of the endoscopist is to shorten and telescope the colon so that the cecum is reached with a limited amount of scope and with minimal patient discomfort. The endoscopist must recognize that obtuse angles are easier to traverse than are acute ones and that it is easier to straighten the bowel first and then advance, rather than vice versa.

INSERTION TECHNIQUES

Anus and Rectum

The area of the anus and perineum is carefully inspected before a gentle digital examination of the rectum. This approach serves several purposes. Any external abnormalities, such as protruding hemorrhoids or fistulae, that may be of clinical significance can be recognized. The bimanual digital rectal examination may uncover prostatic or gynecologic disease or a rectal or cecal lesion previously unsuspected. Determining the adequacy of the bowel preparation as well as preparing and relaxing the anal sphincter for insertion of the endoscope are also accomplished.

The distal 5-10 cm of the colonscopic tip is well lubricated with surgical jelly before insertion. Lubricant may be applied to the scope and around the anus during the examination. The index finger of the right hand is then placed on the lateral surface of the tip of the colonoscope. The tip is brought in apposition to the anal orifice and is better visualized if an assistant elevates the patient's right buttock (Fig. 51). The tip of the endoscope is then gently inserted with slight pressure of the forefinger on the endoscope. Air is constantly insufflated during insertion to enable the endoscopist to visualize the entire anal canal by dilating it during passage and to keep the instruments lens clear.

During passage through the anal canal, the tip is kept straight. As the tip enters the rectum, the endoscopist flexes the instrument by flexing the left thumb on the up/down control to form a 90-degree angle by the endoscope. Thus, at this point, the tip is directed in an upward position, toward the posterior wall of the rectum (Fig. 52a). The triangular point on the view finder of the endoscope corresponds to the posterior wall of the rectum. It then follows that the left

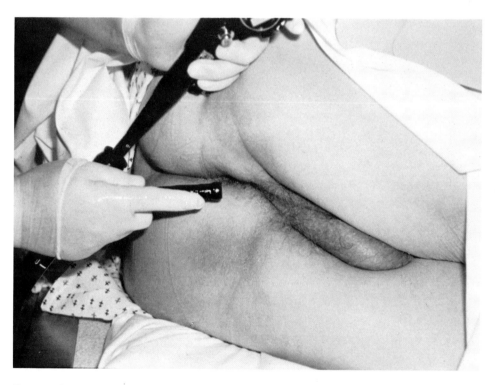

Fig. 51. Insertion of the colonoscope into the anal orifice. The patient's right buttock is elevated by the back of the operator's left hand as the tip of the instrument is being inserted with the right hand.

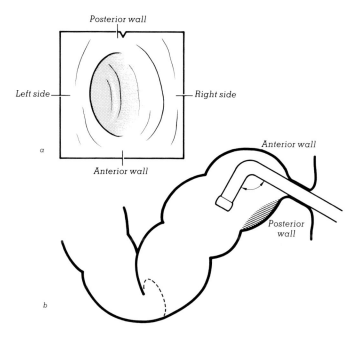

Fig. 52. a: *Anatomic positions in the rectum.* **b:** *Examination of the rectum by right-angle flexion of the colonoscope. The shaded area represents a blind area on the posterior wall of the distal rectum.*

lateral rectal wall is on the operator's left (as viewed through the eyepiece), the right wall is on his right and the anterior wall is downward.

The posterior wall immediately inside the anal canal is easily missed and should be examined by flexing the tip of the instrument (by flexing the left thumb on the up/down control) and pulling the instrument gently toward the anal sphincter (Fig. 52b). Because the patient is in the left lateral recumbent position, fecal fluid may collect along the left lateral rectal wall and hide polypoid lesions. It is important to aspirate completely any such collection.

Complete visualization of the rectal wall is accomplished with a combination of flexion of the tip of the colonoscope and rotation of the endoscope along its long axis, controlled by the right hand. The rectal lumen is relatively large, and the entire circumference must be examined in a systematic fashion. This examination may be best accomplished by advancing the endoscope to the rectosigmoid junction and then slowly withdrawing it to the anal canal with a continuous spiral motion of the tip of the colonoscope. It is important not to overinflate the rectum because this causes patient discomfort and may cause the rectosigmoid angle to become too acute and thus difficult to traverse.

Rectosigmoid Junction

After careful inspection of the rectum, the tip of the instrument is advanced 2-3 cm beyond the rectosigmoid fold and, at the same time, turned slightly to the right. The tip is then flexed and gently pulled caudad. This maneuver will cause the endoscope to pull the fold toward the endoscopist ("hooking the fold") (Fig. 53). The operator continues to exert gentle pressure until the sigmoid lumen comes into view, at which time the instrument is advanced. This maneuver straightens the rectosigmoid angle and allows the endoscopist relatively easy entrance into the sigmoid colon. This approach avoids sharp blind angles and a large amount of air insufflation. It is important not to push the tip of the instrument into the mucosa of the rectosigmoid angle. (There should be no "red out" during this maneuver; if there is, it is being done incorrectly.)

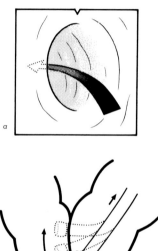

Fig. 53. a: *Advancement beyond the rectosigmoid fold.* **b:** *"Hooking the fold" by flexion and caudad pull.*

Sigmoid and Descending Colon

The instrument is best advanced through the sigmoid colon by pulling back whenever resistance is encountered and by moving the tip gently until the lumen or its direction is determined. The lumen should be followed without attempting to impose a pattern of advancement, such as an alpha maneuver. An attempt should be made to shorten the sigmoid colon, as the operator traverses it, to prevent stretching of the bowel and the mesentery and loss of length of the endoscope later during the procedure. This is accomplished by to and fro motions of the endoscope interspersed with advancement. (This maneuver is described later as the "jiggling" technique.) The tip of the endoscope is thus advanced to the junction of the sigmoid colon and descending colon and usually makes an "N" pattern (Fig. 54). The angle at this junction is widened by pulling the instrument back toward the endoscopist and slightly straightening the tip (Figs. 55 and 56).

Thus, the N pattern becomes a sine wave, and gently pulling the instrument toward the endoscopist transmits tension from the sigmoid colon to the tip of the endoscope as the sigmoid is straightened. The tip of the endoscope is then in position to progress up the descending colon.

If the endoscope forms an alpha loop or reverse alpha loop while advancing through the sigmoid colon (referring to the Greek letter alpha), this loop should be removed when the tip of the endoscope reaches the splenic flexure or proximal descending colon (Fig. 57). This maneuver is accomplished by pulling back the endoscope and turning it in a clockwise rotation (to remove an alpha loop) and a counterclockwise or clockwise rotation (to remove a reverse alpha loop) with the right hand.

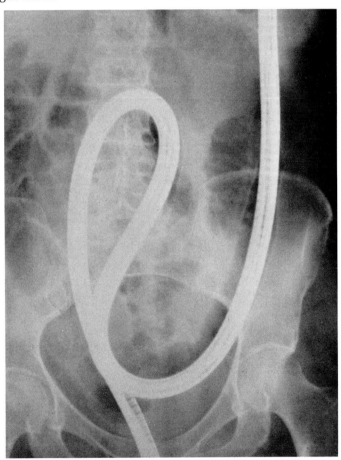

Fig. 54. An N-shaped sigmoid and descending colon. The colonoscope is pulled back as soon as the tip reaches the splenic flexure. The sigmoid is shortened and straightened by telescoping the colon.

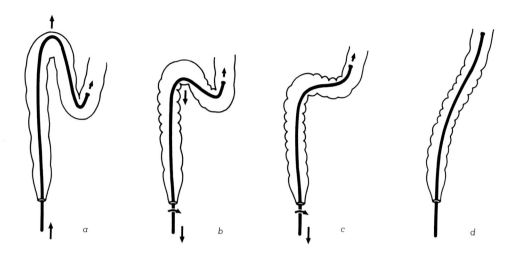

Fig. 55.
a: Colonoscope inserted to the junction of the sigmoid and descending colon, stretching the sigmoid loop and mesentery, resulting in an N-shaped pattern.
b: Angle between sigmoid and descending colon widened by pulling back the instrument and slowly turning to the right, producing a sine-wave configuration of the sigmoid.
c: By pulling back and slowly turning to the right, the angle is widened further, and the sigmoid becomes straight.
d: Advancing the colonoscope through the straightened sigmoid colon.

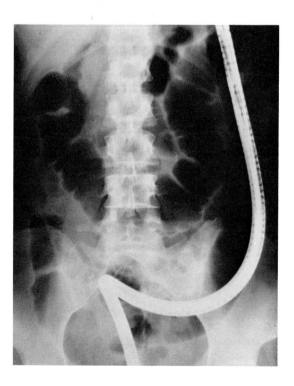

Fig. 56. A J-shaped sigmoid and descending colon. The sigmoid colon may be shortened, usually secondary to resection or advanced diverticulosis.

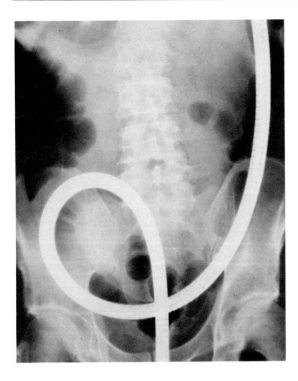

Fig. 57. *An alpha-shaped sigmoid and descending colon. When the colonscope reaches the proximal descending colon, it must be turned to the right and pulled back. This maneuver straightens and shortens the sigmoid before the instrument is advanced further.*

As the technique of an endoscopist improves, this stretching of the sigmoid colon may be avoided by rotating clockwise along the axis of the endoscope and pulling back toward the operator as the operator advances through the sigmoid colon (Fig. 58a and 58b) (see page 61, "Right Turn Shortening Technique").

If the operator reaches the junction of the sigmoid colon and descending colon and a long loop has been formed with an acute angle (Fig. 59a), it may be impossible to advance to the descending colon. In this situation, the endoscope should be withdrawn to the midsigmoid colon to release the tension; the sigmoid loop may then be rotated in a counterclockwise direction (Fig. 59b). Thus, an alpha-loop pattern will be formed (see Fig. 57), which will widen the angle at this junction, and the endoscope will easily advance into the descending colon (Fig. 59c). After the tip is advanced into the proximal descending colon (splenic flexure), the alpha loop may be removed by rotating clockwise and pulling the instrument caudad, toward the operator (Fig. 59d,e).

Any loop that is formed while the scope is advanced through the sigmoid colon and descending colon should be removed before reaching the proximal descending colon to minimize patient discomfort. While pulling the endoscope back toward the endoscopist to straighten the colon (Fig. 60), some lumen must be kept in view at all times and inflated air aspirated. The view should not be "reddened out" or blanched by turning the tip into the bowel wall.

Various combinations of the following techniques are used for traversing the sigmoid colon:

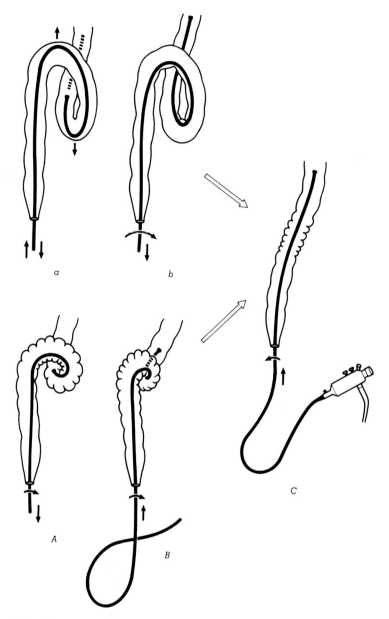

Fig. 58.

a: Forming a reverse alpha loop by stretching the sigmoid and its mesentery.

b: Removing the reverse alpha loop by counterclockwise or clockwise rotation and pulling back on the colonoscope on reaching the splenic flexure.

A: Clockwise rotation for advancing through the junction of the sigmoid and descending colon (right-turn shortening technique).

B: Further advancing, rotating clockwise and pulling back straightens the sigmoid colon.

C: Both techniques produce a straight sigmoid colon.

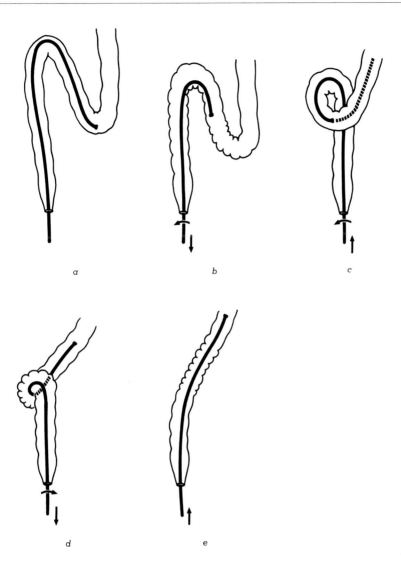

Fig. 59.
a: Long loop with acute angle at junction of the sigmoid and descending colon.
b: Instrument withdrawn to the midsigmoid colon, leaving a free segment of sigmoid for subsequent rotation.
c: Sigmoid loop rotated counterclockwise, producing an alpha loop pattern.
d: Alpha loop removed by rotating clockwise and withdrawing the instrument.
e: Straightened sigmoid colon.

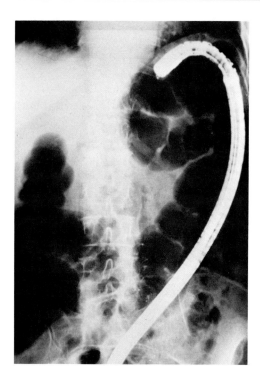

Fig. 60. A colonoscope is advanced to the splenic flexure and left transverse colon after straightening the sigmoid colon.

Direct Insertion Technique

This method involves straightforward insertion of the endoscope while the sigmoid lumen is visualized directly. The endoscope is advanced by performing a simple to and fro motion, keeping the sigmoid lumen inflated for a distance of several centimeters. The endoscope is advanced with the oncoming lumen in view.

Pull-Back and Rotation Technique

This method is best used for short, straight sigmoid colons or those that have been partially resected. If the lumen is not visualized, the endoscope should be withdrawn and/or rotated until the lumen again comes into view. In this manner, the operator can easily advance to the descending colon. This principle can be applied to any part of the colon.

Slide-by the Mucosa Technique

Although the sigmoid lumen is not visualized directly, knowing the direction that it takes enables the operator to "slide by" the mucosa, thus advancing the instrument through an acutely angulated segment of colon. When an acute angulation is encountered in the sigmoid colon, it may be overcome by advancing the endoscope with the tip of the instrument partially in contact with the colonic mucosa. Thus, the mucosa slides by rapidly over the tip of the endoscope for a short distance without encountering much resistance until the lumen once again comes into view. If the colonic mucosa blanches during this maneuver, this reaction indicates that the endoscope is being pressed into the colonic wall at a right angle, and perforation may occur. The endoscope should then be withdrawn, and the direction of the lumen should be reestablished. The slide-by technique is used only in short segments of colon, usually near an angle. It should not be applied to cases of diverticulosis, inflammatory bowel disease or if extrinsic fixation or adhesions exist. While using this technique, if the lumen is not seen, the scope should be pulled back gently without changing the direction of the tip. If the lumen still is not seen, the maneuver may be repeated as long as resistance is not encountered and the mucosa is not reddened out. The slide-by maneuver should not be applied continuously but, rather, in short, successive, in and out motions. During the maneuver, the operator should expect the endoscope to advance in direct proportion to the length being inserted. If this is not the case, the tip of the endoscope is stretching the bowel wall and the mesentery.

Abdominal Manipulations

To advance the endoscope through the midportion of a redundant sigmoid colon and to concomitantly avoid stretching the bowel mesentery, gentle extra-abdominal pressure of an assistant's hand over the left lower quadrant will enable the bowel to be maintained in a straightened position. If the colon is being stretched while the operator advances to the proximal sigmoid, the endoscope should be flexed (with flexion of the left thumb) and pulled back toward the operator. At the same time, an assistant's hand pressed down over the left lower quadrant or upper to midabdomen will fix the sigmoid colon and prevent bowing of the loop.

Right-Turn Shortening Technique

This technique is useful in traversing short to moderately redundant sigmoid colons. It is not an easy maneuver to master, and more redundant sigmoid colons require an experienced endoscopist's hand. This maneuver cannot be performed if the procedure is being done by two operators. The instrument is advanced progressively into the sigmoid colon by following the lumen. Each sigmoid fold that comes into view is hooked and gently brought back toward the endoscopist while the endoscope is gradually rotated clockwise to the right. When the tip of the instrument reaches the junction of the sigmoid colon and the descending colon, the angle between the endoscope tip and long axis of the instrument should be slightly greater than 90 degrees (closer to a sine wave). Then, by determining the direction of the lumen and turning the endoscope to the right, the descending colon is entered. Because of the constant clockwise rotation and withdrawal of the endoscope, which shortens the bowel, the endoscope outside of the patient becomes looped (alpha loop). When the mid- to proximal descending colon is reached, the operator can rotate the instrument counterclockwise without losing distance or encountering resistance. This observation implies that the scope is straight.

Jiggling Technique (rapid to and fro motion)

This method may be used when it is desirable to have the colon shortened and straightened. The endoscope is withdrawn several centimeters (removing stretching of the bowel) and then, without advancing the instrument, the tip is put through a series of rapid to and fro motions that telescope, shorten, and straighten the colon. This technique can be used whenever the endoscope does not advance, the mesentery is being stretched or unusual resistance is encountered during insertion.

Splenic Flexure

With the bowel completely straightened, the length of the inserted instrument to the splenic flexure measures about 40-50 cm in length from the anal verge. At this point, the operator must determine the direction of the transverse colon. The endoscope is then flexed to form a 90-degree angle between the tip and the long axis of the endoscope, and the endoscope is pulled gently toward the operator. This maneuver will flatten the peak of the splenic flexure. If the tip of the endoscope is flexed to 180 degrees, the insertion power will be transmitted to the level of flexion rather than to the tip, thus stretching the splenic flexure to the diaphragm rather than advancing the tip into the transverse colon. Advancing into the transverse colon is often best accomplished by visualizing the upper portion of the lumen so that the tip is not acutely flexed (Fig. 61). Gentle to and fro motion is necessary to flatten the angle between the descending colon and the transverse colon and to keep the sigmoid straight. Forceful withdrawal of the flexed endoscope at this level can injure the spleen.

During the maneuver, it is important to keep the sigmoid colon straight so that insertion power is easily transmitted to the tip of the instrument, thus

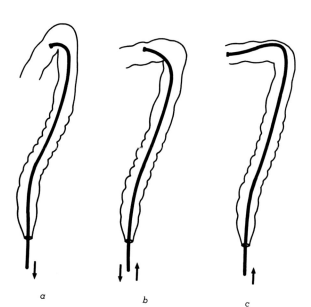

Fig. 61.
a: Colonoscope advanced to the splenic flexure, flexed and gently pulled back. A colonoscope in the sigmoid and descending colon should be straight when it passes the splenic flexure.
b: Flattening of the splenic flexure peak by gentle to and fro motions, and widening of the angle with the tip of the colonoscope flexed.
c: Advancing into the left transverse colon.

a   b   c

keeping the patient comfortable. Counterclockwise rotation of the endoscope should be avoided (this usually results in making a loop of the sigmoid).

While traversing the splenic flexure, in patients with a redundant sigmoid, a straightened colon can be maintained in that condition by external abdominal manipulation or insertion of a splinting device.

Transverse Colon

The transverse colon is easily identified by its characteristic triangular folds. The transmitted aortic pulsation is also seen and felt as the transverse colon is entered. While passing to the left transverse colon, the endoscope should be kept close to the inferior aspect of the colon. In this way, the operator will be able to visualize the entire lumen and conserve scope length.

As the midtransverse colon is reached, the tip is flexed slightly upward toward the right transverse colon. At this point, suction is applied, and paradoxical advancement to the hepatic flexure is commonly achieved by pulling the endoscope back toward the operator (Figs. 62 and 63). During this maneuver, the patient should be maintained on his or her left side because gravity helps to keep the bowel telescoped on the instrument. If the patient is supine, or on his or her right side, this advantage may be lost. After this maneuver, to prevent rebowing of the transverse colon, right-sided pressure and traction are applied by the palm of the assistant's hand on the left midabdomen. The patient's back is simultaneouly supported to prevent him or her from rolling into the supine position.

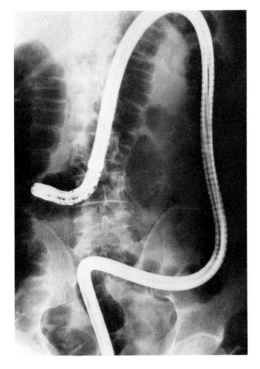

Fig. 62. *A colonoscope is advanced to the mid and right transverse colon by aspirating intraluminal air and pulling back the instrument.*

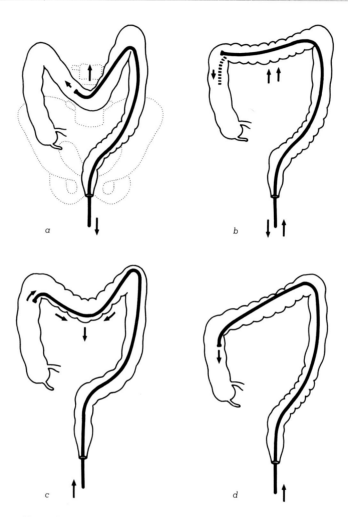

Fig. 63.

a: As the midtransverse colon is reached, the tip is flexed upward by turning the control knob downward. Suction is applied, and the instrument is withdrawn. This maneuver leads to paradoxical advancement to the hepatic flexure.

b: The assistant's upward pressure on the transverse colon prevents a U-shaped configuration and allows the operator to advance to the hepatic flexure and beyond.

c: The tip is advanced to the ascending colon, and the instrument is withdrawn. The transverse colon is straightened.

d: Paradoxical withdrawal of the instrument may occur if it is inserted into the ascending colon, before the transverse colon is straightened.

In patients with extremely redundant transverse colons in whom the transverse colon cannot be properly telescoped, the instrument has to be advanced to the hepatic flexure with some stretching of the transverse colon. The endoscope will have a "U"-shaped appearance. Again, an assistant's hand may help prevent major stretching and serve to direct force toward the tip of the instrument and not to the base of the U. When the instrument forms a U-shape in the transverse colon, it is necessary to advance the tip to the midascending colon before pulling back and attempting to straighten the transverse colon (Figs. 64a and 64b). If the operator tries to straighten the transverse colon unsuccessfully, by pulling the scope back before the tip is in the ascending colon, further attempts to advance the tip will result in paradoxical withdrawal (Fig. 63c). At this point, the operator must resume gentle forward insertion of the scope until the ascending colon is well entered.

Hepatic Flexure, Ascending Colon and Cecum

Even for a skilled operator, the hepatic flexure may be one of the most difficult anatomic areas to pass. The optimum goal is to achieve, fluoroscopically, a figure "7" with the endoscope when it has advanced to the cecum (Fig. 64e). This goal is accomplished when the colon has been completely straightened and is well telescoped. Nearly all colonoscopies should end this way, with minimal patient discomfort. If the transverse colon forms a large U and the right colon forms a clockwise internal spiral (Fig. 64b), it is almost impossible to change the configuration to the ideal figure 7 before reaching the cecum or the proximal ascending colon. This configuration can cause patient discomfort. To prevent such discomfort, the operator should keep withdrawing the scope and aspirate inflated air frequently. A splinting device and abdominal manipulation should be helpful in such cases.

A gamma loop (referring to the Greek letter gamma) of the transverse colon is sometimes formed unintentionally (Figs. 64c and 64d). Stretching the transverse colon may be as uncomfortable to the patient as stretching the sigmoid colon. However, having a gamma loop in the transverse colon is occasionally advantageous since widening of the angle of the hepatic flexure serves to facilitate advancement to the ascending colon and the cecum. During the formation of the gamma loop, the operator often is not able to visualize the lumen completely. Also, during withdrawal, the instrument tends to slip out rapidly, and thus there may be many blind areas in the transverse colon. After the tip of the instrument is in the cecum, the gamma loop should be removed and the transverse colon straightened by either clockwise or counterclockwise rotation, depending upon which way the loop is crossed. This maneuver should be carried out with fluoroscopic guidance. Again, occasionally, the redundant right-side colon will form an internal right spiral (Fig. 64b). The normal hepatocecal axis (imagine one connecting the hepatic flexure with the cecal valve) will transect this spiral formation. This configuration causes much patient discomfort and is seen more frequently with novice endoscopists. Once this configuration is

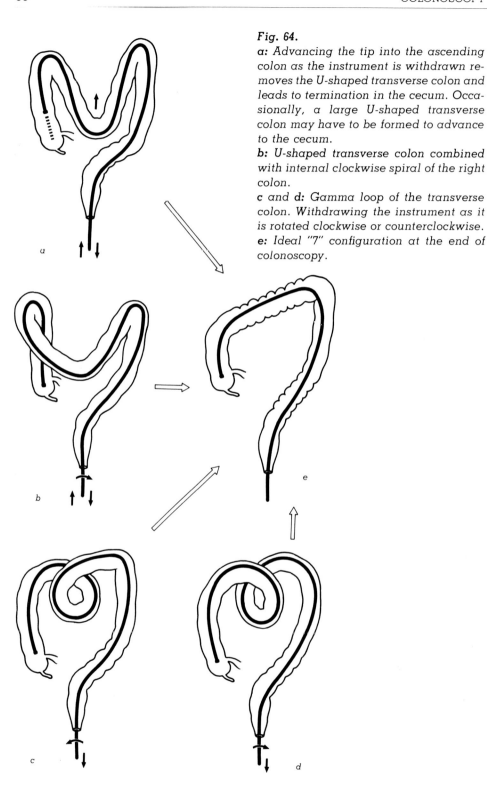

Fig. 64.

a: Advancing the tip into the ascending colon as the instrument is withdrawn removes the U-shaped transverse colon and leads to termination in the cecum. Occasionally, a large U-shaped transverse colon may have to be formed to advance to the cecum.

b: U-shaped transverse colon combined with internal clockwise spiral of the right colon.

c and **d:** Gamma loop of the transverse colon. Withdrawing the instrument as it is rotated clockwise or counterclockwise.

e: Ideal "7" configuration at the end of colonoscopy.

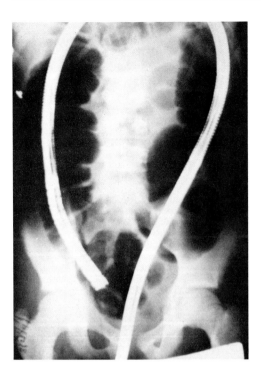

Fig. 65. A colonoscope is fully inserted in the cecum, thus straightening a redundant sigmoid and transverse colon.

formed, it is better to reach the cecum and then withdraw than to attempt to straighten it.

   Once the colon has been straightened, reaching the cecum by straightforward advancement is usually accomplished without difficulty (Fig. 65). The operator usually can ascertain his or her position using fluoroscopy or by tapping gently over the right lower quadrant with the right hand. With the latter maneuver, while looking through the endoscope viewpiece, the operator will see a bouncing of the cecum around the scope tip. If the operator is not in the cecum, no movement will be observed. One other method for determining the position of the endoscope, in a thin patient, is to temporarily dim the lights and observe the position of the red glow of the tip.

Ileocecal Junction (Valve) and Entrance into the Terminal Ileum

As stated, the appendiceal orifice is readily located by identifying the junction of the three taeniae of the colon. While occasionally this junction is the true apex of the cecum, usually the appendiceal opening is seen medially and superiorly by enlargement of the right saccule between the anterior and posterior taeniae. This feature is important in locating the ileocecal valve, which lies 4-6 cm distal to the appendiceal orifice and about 15 degrees anterior to the medial taenia. The two lips of the valve are oriented transversely at the junction

of the cecum and ascending colon, and although they cannot always be identified separately, entrance into the terminal ileum is gained by first locating
both lips of the valve. The tip of the endoscope is then advanced past both lips
(Fig. 66a), then flexed and brought to the level of the slit while applying a slight
counterclockwise rotation to the shaft (Fig. 66b). This maneuver causes the
upper lip to be lifted by the tip of the instrument, and the entrance to the
terminal ileum can thus be visualized (Fig. 66c). It may have to be repeated
several times until the terminal ileum is finally entered. Of the three types of
valves, type I is the most difficult to traverse. Once the terminal ileum is entered, one can usually advance the scope at least 25 cm into the bowel without
difficulty.

The ileocecal junction is not seen in the en face view until the upper lip of the
ileocecal valve is lifted by the tip of the endoscope.

The ileocecal valve may appear as one of three basic forms (Fig. 66). The first
resembles a thin mucosal slit or very thin, tightly closed lips. This variety is
encountered in approximately 22% of cases. The second type has a more prominent and thicker appearance. This variety is much more common, seen in about
67% of cases. The third type has an oval shape and is the thickest. It is the least
common form, occurring in 11% of cases.

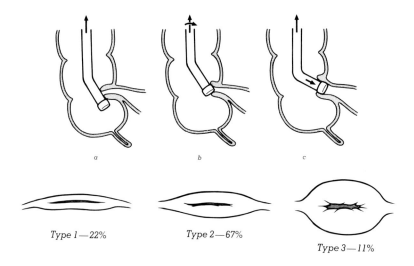

Type 1—22%   Type 2—67%

Type 3—11%

Fig. 66. Top: Technique for inserting a colonscope into the terminal
ileum. **a:** The tip of the instrument is advanced beyond the ileocecal
valve. **b:** The tip is flexed and brought back to the level of the lips.
c: Slight counterclockwise rotation of the shaft lifts the upper lip and
allows for insertion into the terminal ileum.
Bottom: Types of ileocecal valve. Type 1, thin mucosal slit valve;
type 2, prominent, thick valve; type 3, thick, oval valve.

SPLINTING DEVICE (SLIDING TUBE)

To prevent bowing of a redundant sigmoid colon during passage of the splenic flexure, after the splenic flexure has been passed, two stiffening devices have been used. The first is an internal splint passed through the biopsy channel of the colonoscope. This splint stiffens the flexible scope to a small degree. Because of its minimal effect in maintaining rigidity, and possible damage to the colonoscope, this device is rarely used today.

The more commonly used aid is the external splinting device. It is a 40-cm long, semi-rigid, tapered tube through which the colonoscope can be inserted (Fig. 67). The primary function of this device is to shorten and straighten the sigmoid colon and to prevent bowing of the sigmoid so that the scope can be advanced more easily into the transverse colon and the cecum.

This device can be used in any situation where the sigmoid colon can be straightened easily and safely.

In my experience, examination time can be markedly shortened and patient discomfort minimized. In addition, using this device in more than 2,000 patients, we have not experienced any complications. However, this device should be used cautiously and with full understanding of its principles.

This device can also be used in retrieving multiple polyps from the transverse colon and right colon (see Fig. 267, Chapter 15). By repeated insertion of the scope through a splinted sigmoid colon, the hazard of renegotiating a difficult and redundant sigmoid can be avoided. For insertion of the splinting device, only the long scope can be used. After it is in position, a short instrument can be passed through the splint.

This technique for inserting the splinting device (stiffening device) is as follows:

The long colonoscope is passed through the device before it is inserted (Figs. 68 and 69). It is then rested at the proximal portion of the instrument. The colonoscope is next inserted in the usual fashion. If a difficult redundant sigmoid colon is encountered, the alpha maneuver can be performed. This maneuver widens the angle at the junction of the sigmoid colon and descending colon and allows for easier insertion of the colonoscope. When under fluoroscopic

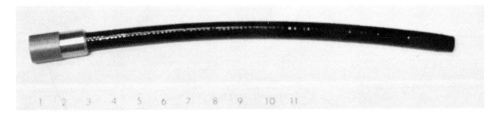

Fig. 67. Splinting device or sliding tube (length, 40 cm).

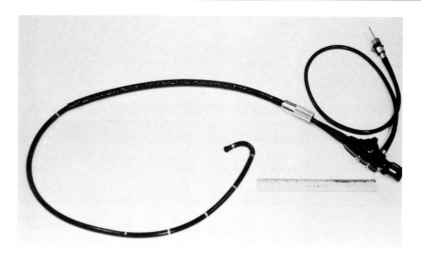

Fig. 68. A splinting device is placed over the shaft of the colonoscope before insertion.

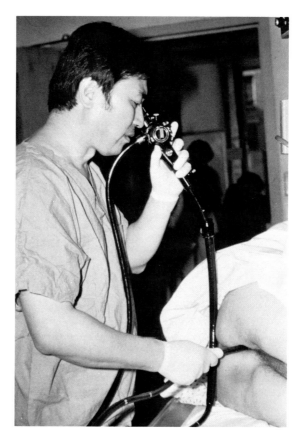

Fig. 69. A colonoscope is introduced with the
patient in the left lateral recumbent position. A
splinting device is placed over the shaft of the
instrument.

control the splenic flexure is identified or the left transverse colon is reached, the endoscope is gently withdrawn and turned to the right so that the alpha loop is released and the sigmoid colon is straightened (Fig. 70). To maintain this position, the splinting device is inserted. The tip of the splint, which is slightly tapered, is well lubricated and then gently inserted into the rectum using a screwlike motion with the thumb and forefinger of the left hand. At the same time, the right hand fixes the colonoscope, so that it does not move with the splint (Fig. 71). Under fluoroscopic control, the splint is then gently advanced through the sigmoid colon until it reaches the mid- to proximal descending colon (Figs. 73 and 74). The tip of the splint should not be advanced over the distal flexion joint of the instrument. If this movement occurs, not only will it be impossible to flex the instrument fully, but the cable may be severed as well.

The splinting device should never be inserted forcefully. If any resistance is encountered, further insertion of the splint should not be carried out, especially in patients with diverticular disease, stricture or status after several abdominal procedures.

With the splint in place, the scope is then advanced through the remainder of the colon to the cecum (Figs. 75–80).

Once the endoscopist becomes proficient with the use of the splinting device, fluoroscopy will be necessary only when resistance is encountered.

In cases where an alpha loop must be formed to allow for further insertion of the colonoscope, the sigmoid loop may become extremely bowed. This bowing prevents the proper turn to the left necessary to obtain the alpha configuration. To avoid this potential difficulty, the scope is pulled back, and the rectum and the lower sigmoid colon are straightened. The splinting device is then inserted, under fluoroscopic control, past the rectosigmoid junction. The splint keeps this anatomic flexure straight and allows for the proper formation of the alpha loop (Fig. 72). The splinting device is then pulled back to the rectum or the outside and reintroduced to the mid-descending colon after the scope is straightened.

In cases where several polyps or pieces of segmentally excised polyps must be retrieved from the transverse colon and the right colon after polypectomy, the splinting device is inserted to the proximal descending colon and is left in place to maintain this position. Polyps can then be retrieved individually from the transverse colon and the right colon without having to renegotiate a difficult or redundant sigmoid colon.

ADVANTAGES OF THE SPLINTING DEVICE

1. Prevents bowing of a redundant sigmoid colon
2. Straightens the rectosigmoid junction
3. Straightens the sigmoid-descending colon junction
4. Allows easy retrieval of right-sided colonic polyps after polypectomy

DISADVANTAGES OF THE SPLINTING DEVICE

1. Must be used under fluoroscopic control in most circumstances
2. Cannot be inserted if there is appreciable anal or sigmoid narrowing
3. May cause bleeding or "autopolypectomy" of polyps in the sigmoid colon
4. May, in rare instances, cause colonic perforation if not used cautiously

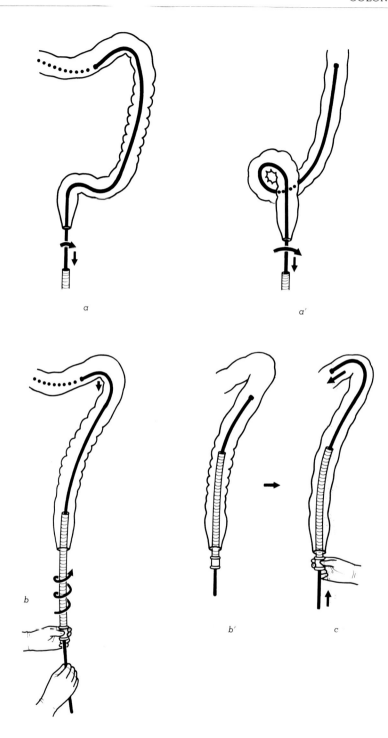

a

a'

b

b'

c

Fig. 70.

a: A colonoscope is advanced to the left transverse colon and pulled back to straighten the sigmoid and descending colon before insertion of the splinting device.

a': Formation of an alpha loop to overcome a redundant sigmoid colon.

b: After the sigmoid and descending colon is straightened, the splinting device is inserted by slow rotation over the colonoscope under fluoroscopic control. If fluoroscopy is not used during insertion of the splint, there should be no resistance during its introduction.

b': When the colonoscope reaches the splenic flexure or left transverse colon, the loop is released by withdrawing the instrument and turning clockwise (right). The splint is inserted completely under fluoroscopic control.

c: A colonoscope is advanced through the transverse colon with a splinted sigmoid.

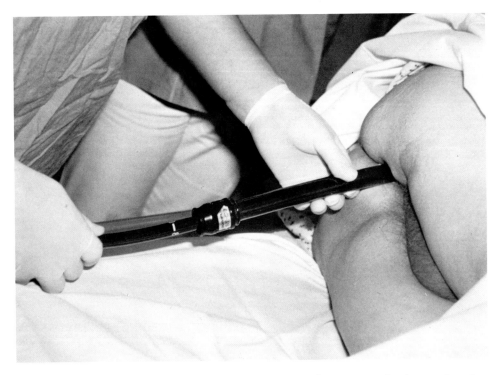

Fig. 71. A splinting device is gently inserted into the anus and advanced under fluoroscopic control. The right hand holds the colonoscope in position.

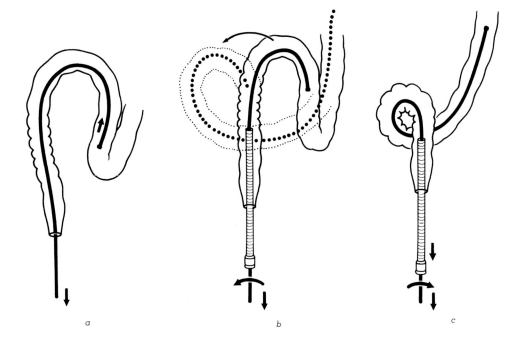

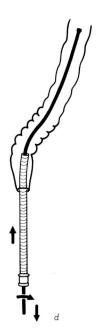

Fig. 72.

a: Bowing of the sigmoid loop prevents the left turn necessary to produce an alpha configuration. The colonoscope is pulled back toward the rectum.

b: A splinting device is inserted, under fluoroscopic control past the rectosigmoid junction. An alpha loop is formed by counterclockwise rotation.

c: The splinting device is pulled back to the rectum, and the alpha loop is removed by clockwise rotation.

d: The sigmoid is straightened, and the instrument is advanced.

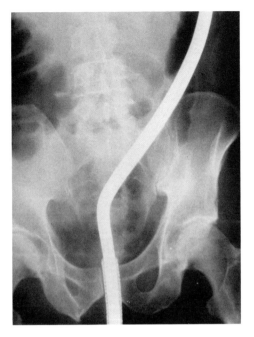

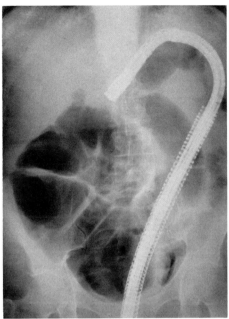

Fig. 73. X-ray film with the splint partially inserted and the sigmoid colon being straightened.

Fig. 74. The splint is advanced to the proximal descending colon. The splenic flexure is hooked, and the sigmoid is completely straight.

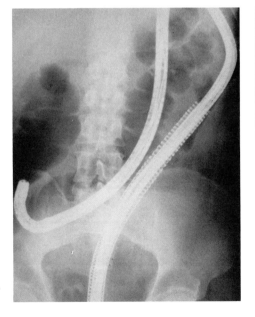

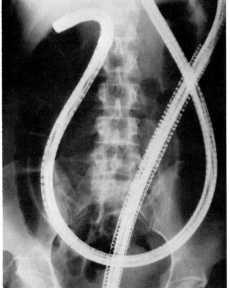

Fig. 75. A colonoscope is advanced through the transverse colon to the hepatic flexure. A splinting device keeps the sigmoid shortened and straight.

Fig. 76. A redundant loop of transverse colon. The tip of the colonoscope can be advanced past the hepatic flexure only by pushing the instrument.

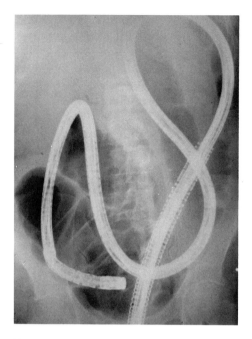

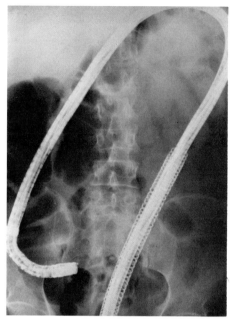

Fig. 77. *Pushing the colonoscope allows it to advance to the cecum.*

Fig. 78. *The colonoscope is advanced to the cecum after the redundant transverse and sigmoid colon is straightened. A splint is in place.*

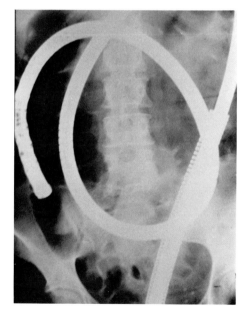

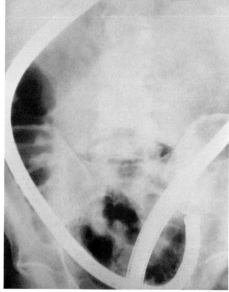

Fig. 79. *A redundant transverse colon forming a gamma loop.*

Fig. 80. *After pulling back the colonoscope and the splint, the loop is straightened and the instrument advances into the terminal ileum.*

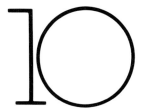

Endoscopic Diagnosis of Colonic Diseases

DIVERTICULAR DISEASE

Colonic diverticular disease is a common lesion in the urban areas of the western world. This disease represents acquired mucosal herniations that project through the bowel wall. The sigmoid colon is affected 95% of the time. At least 40% of patients over the age of 70 have diverticula demonstrated by barium roentgenograms. The herniations are due to elevated intraluminal colonic pressure, areas of weakness in the bowel wall or a combination of both. Manometric studies show a high pressure zone in the sigmoid colon.

Complications of diverticulosis include diverticulitis and hemorrhage. Diverticulitis develops in 12%-50% of patients with diverticulosis, many of whom have no clinical history. Additional gross and histologic changes include thickening of the circular and longitudinal muscles of the colon wall and redundant-appearing mucosae and diverticular lumen that range from 1 mm to 1.0 cm in diameter. Since diverticulosis commonly coexists with other benign and malignant diseases of the colon, colonoscopy is frequently done and unsuspected lesions are often encountered.

Endoscopic Features of Diverticular Disease

The patient with diverticular disease is more difficult to examine with the colonoscope because of spasm, a narrowed lumen with prominent mucosal folds, fixation and angulation of the colon, and diverticuli which one may confuse with a luminal opening (Figs. 81, 82).

77

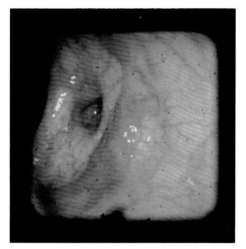 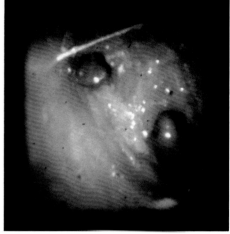

Fig. 81. Solitary diverticulum of the sig-   *Fig. 82.* Several wide-mouthed diverticu-
moid colon.   lar orifices in the sigmoid. The colonic
                                                  lumen bends to the right.

A characteristic feature of diverticular disease of the sigmoid is marked
mucosal redundancy with folds of the mucosa filling the lumen of the colon and
contributing to the narrowing caused by muscular thickening. Fixation and
angulation of the bowel may be due to pericolic fibrosis with extensive pericolic
and mesenteric fat tissue. A diverticulum is often plugged with a large fecalith
on endoscopic examination. Diverticular orifices are easier to identify on insertion of the scope during the stretching of the colonic mucosa than at the time of
withdrawal of the scope (Fig. 83).

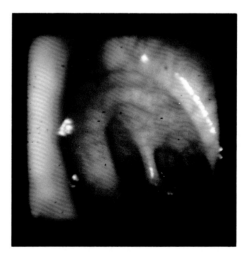

Fig. 83. Extremely large diverticular
orifices with narrowing of the sigmoid.

Indications for Colonoscopy in Patients with Diverticulosis

A barium enema remains the most useful means of demonstrating diverticulosis, but this procedure should be supplemented by colonoscopy in the following situations:

1. When a polyp, carcinoma or both coexist with diverticulosis
2. When the differential diagnosis lies between diverticulitis and carcinoma
3. When diverticulosis and inflammatory bowel disease coexist in the same segment of bowel (the former is localized inflammation with or without purulent drainage and without mucosal inflammation; the latter is ulcerative or granulomatous colitis within segments of diverticulosis)
4. When there is overt or occult intestinal bleeding

Colonoscopy is usually of great value in establishing the diagnosis in these circumstances.

Technique

The most common location of diverticulosis and diverticulitis is the sigmoid colon.

Diverticular strictures may not allow an adult colonoscope to pass beyond a narrowed area; a pediatric scope should be used in such cases. Force should never be applied to direct the endoscope through these segments. It is very difficult to differentiate a colonic stricture from severe spasm. If a barium enema revealed diverticulosis and narrowing of the colon, glucagon or dicyclomine administered before or during the procedure may facilitate examination by relaxing the spasm. Care must be taken when spasm is present to prevent the insufflated air from accumulating in the proximal colon, which would lead to severe abdominal pain after the examination. To avoid this potential sequela, all the air is aspirated while the endoscope is withdrawn.

In response to insertion of the colonoscope, the diverticular colon may become hyperactive and spastic. Endoscopic progression may be slowed because of frequent contractions. As the examination proceeds, the irritability may subside, but a parenteral antispasmodic agent may be required (e.g., glucagon or dicyclomine) to facilitate and maintain patient comfort.

Forceful insertion is never advised in examining a diverticular colon since injury and perforation occur easily. Since novice endoscopists may attempt to traverse a diverticular orifice, believing it to be lumen, it is important that they accurately determine the direction of the lumen before proceeding.

Diverticulitis

With acute active diverticulitis, treatment of the bowel disease precedes elective colonoscopic evaluation. After the attack subsides, a barium enema is obtained to exclude carcinoma, obstruction or a sealed perforation, which may require early surgery.

If there is no clinical or radiologic evidence of diverticulitis or other complications (perforation, fistula, obstruction, extensive bleeding), endoscopic evaluation may be done. As mentioned, this procedure can confirm the original diagnosis and exclude a coexisting carcinoma or other inflammatory disease. Excluding these sequelae allows more leisure treatment of the primary disease or a possible recurrent attack.

Not infrequently, an acute clinical picture dictates the need for surgical intervention. Although there are many operations from which to choose, a colostomy is frequently done, sometimes along with a sigmoid resection, depending on local findings. A barium enema and colonoscopy then allow examination of defunctionalized left colon. Coexisting pathology, particularly cancer, can be excluded. Colonoscopy may be performed 7-10 days after a surgical procedure. An endoscope can be introduced rectally or via colostomy. If active diverticular disease is present, repeat examinations may be necessary until the inflammatory process subsides. Repeat examinations may also determine the optimal time for a planned resection of the colon.

Chronic or subacute diverticulitis is characterized endoscopically by areas of narrowing and edematous mucosa with or without erythema. A few patients who have diverticular symptoms and diverticulosis on barium enema may not show inflammatory mucosal changes. This clinical picture may be due to resolution of the inflammatory process, but the endoscopist should carefully examine each diverticular orifice for purulent drainage. There may be few mucosal clues of a pericolic abscess; the evidence may be hidden within fatty tissue. Because such abscesses are small, they may be missed by the barium contrast study. Colonoscopy is important in such cases because it accurately localizes diseased areas and confirms the diagnosis of diverticulitis (Fig. 84).

Diverticular Disease and Carcinoma

Diverticulosis and colonic carcinoma tend to occur in a similar age group, and both lesions can coexist. In our study of 427 patients with colonic carcinoma,

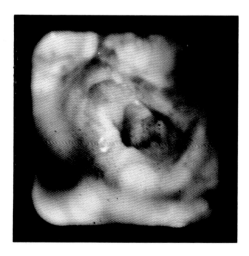

Fig. 84. Diverticulitis with narrowing of the sigmoid. A purulent exudate is seen in the lumen.

102 patients (24%) had coexisting diverticulosis and carcinoma, and one fourth (25%) had both lesions in the descending or sigmoid colon or both (Fig. 85).

Focal narrowing and irregularity of the colon wall due to shortening and thickening of longitudinal and circular muscles may make it difficult to demonstrate coexisting polyps or small carcinomas. The colonoscope sometimes cannot be passed beyond the proximal sigmoid colon because of inflammatory strictures.

Thus, both colonoscopy and barium enema may be necessary to establish the diagnosis of carcinoma with diverticular disease. Even pathologists sometimes have difficulty differentiating between carcinoma with inflammation and diverticulitis with carcinoma.

Diverticular Disease and Inflammatory Bowel Disease

Ulcerative colitis or granulomatous colitis is infrequently associated with diverticular disease. When the latter is found, it is usually associated with granulomatous colitis since this disease is more common among elderly persons. If the mucosa appears granular or ulcerated, a biopsy should be obtained to confirm the diagnosis of inflammatory bowel disease (Fig. 86).

Diverticulosis and Rectal Bleeding

Massive bleeding from the rectum necessitates a full diagnostic work-up, including barium enema and colonoscopy. Selective abdominal angiography may

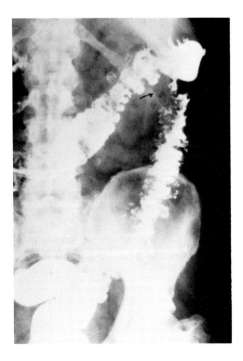

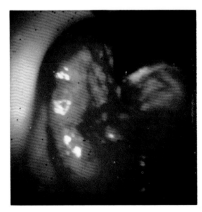

Fig. 85. This patient had evidence of rectal bleeding and left-sided abdominal pain. The barium enema (left) shows diverticulitis with narrowing of the descending colon. A colonoscopic picture of the involved area (right) shows a constricting, ulcerating carcinoma.

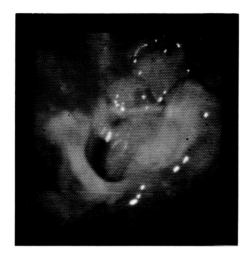

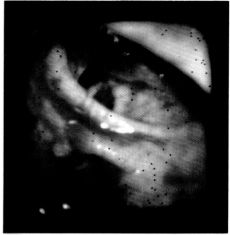

Fig. 86. *A purulent exudate emanates from a diverticulum in a patient with inflammatory bowel disease.*

Fig. 87. *Diverticulosis with blood oozing from a diverticular orifice.*

help, particularly if this procedure is done during active and massive bleeding to localize the bleeding site. In a patient with known diverticulosis, the most likely source of bleeding is from a diverticulum. However, hemangiomas or other vascular lesions also can cause bleeding. Colonoscopy can be performed during the bleeding, but if there is a massive amount of blood, detection of the bleeding site is difficult. It is more useful to perform colonoscopy after bleeding ceases. We have been referred six patients with a known history of diverticular disease and recurrent massive rectal bleeding in whom colonoscopy demonstrated hemangiomas that we believe were the source of blood loss. They were confirmed at surgery. It has previously been reported that rectal bleeding develops in 10%-30% of patients with diverticular disease. The diagnosis of the diverticulum as the source can be made only after all other lesions in the gastrointestinal tract or a bleeding diathesis has been excluded.

In our experience with more than 10,000 colonoscopies in patients with diverticular disease, we have encountered bleeding from a diverticulum only twice (Fig. 87).

The diagnostic evaluation of a patient with diverticulosis and minimal rectal bleeding or occult blood in the stool should include colonoscopy and upper GI endoscopy if the findings of barium studies and upper GI series are negative. Endoscopy is an important adjunct to barium studies and in many cases allows detection of unsuspected lesions.

INFLAMMATORY BOWEL DISEASE

Chronic ulcerative colitis and Crohn's colitis are inflammatory bowel diseases of unknown etiology that initially affect, respectively, the mucosal and submucosal layers, of the bowel wall.

Whereas ulcerative colitis was described over 100 years ago, Crohn's disease was recognized as a distinct disease entity less than 50 years ago. Initially, differentiation between the two diseases seemed clear: each affected different parts of the bowel, each was marked by characteristic pathologic changes and each was easily, if not clearly, discernible from the other. As experience and reports accumulate, and overlap in symptoms, clinical appearance, and disease distribution are described, differentiation at times seems arbitrary.

Chronic Ulcerative Colitis

This disease is an inflammatory process confined to the mucosa and, occasionally, the submucosa. The disease originates in the rectal crypts, with the initial lesion a crypt abscess. Rarely are the deep muscular layers and serosa involved. Coalescence and enlargement of the microabscesses as well as undermining of the mucosa produce a pseudopolyp, which is an ulcerated area surrounding an island of normal mucosa. These changes are nonspecific and can be seen after radiation injury, infection by *Shigella* or gonococci and Crohn's disease of the colon. The pathologic changes in such cases are supported by the clinical features, namely, bloody diarrhea and a purulent discharge. The inflamed mucosa bleeds easily, and because the mucosal membrane is damaged, loss of water and failure to reabsorb salt are possible sequelae. The lack of peritoneal or intra-abdominal signs confirms that the disease is confined to the mucosa or submucosa.

Deep extension and perforation of the colon occur infrequently but may result in stricturing and fibrosis of the bowel wall or, at the other extreme, toxic megacolon.

Endoscopy has substantially improved our ability to diagnose chronic ulcerative colitis and allows the endoscopist to follow pathologic changes. There are many changes in ulcerative colitis, initially consisting of dulling of the submucosal vessels due to edema and tiny mucosal irregularities that may give the surface a granular appearance. Hemorrhage of mucosal and submucosal vessels gives a purpuric appearance to the bowel wall. The initial changes may be subtle, but as the clinical course progresses, the mucosal changes become obvious and marked (Figs. 88, 89).

With active or chronic disease, mucosal erythema becomes manifest. Erosions form larger ulcers, and in some areas the mucosa is friable and bleeds easily when touched by a swab or instrument. The fine reticular pattern of the mucosal vasculature is lost, and the rectal valves may be blunted by inflammation and edema (Fig. 90).

The fine granular pattern becomes irregular and develops into a coarsely granular pattern. Areas of exudate and purulence are present in the mucosa and submucosa; with extension of the ulcer, a pseudopolyp develops. At this stage, there usually is marked spasticity, and the examination must be done with great care. I discontinue further examination if the rectal changes are this severe, fearing perforation of the bowel wall (Figs. 91-93).

Pseudopolyps are more common in chronic disease. They consist of tags of undermined mucosa and granulations or a combination of these abnormalities. Submucosal fibrosis and contracture of the colon may exaggerate the size and

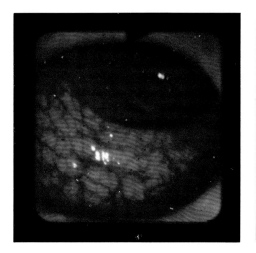 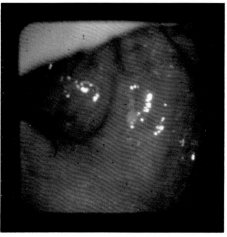

Fig. 88. A patient with repeated episodes of rectal bleeding. Endoscopy revealed hyperemic mucosa (above). Six months later, the endoscopic picture showed ulcerative colitis. In retrospect, the above picture may represent an early stage of inflammatory bowel disease.

Fig. 89. Endoscopic view of markedly edematous mucosa with loss of normal vascular pattern in a patient who eventually had typical ulcerative colitis.

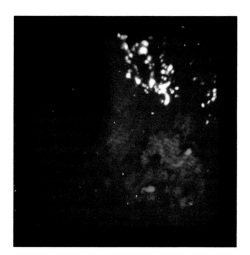

Fig. 90. Early, active ulcerative colitis. Moderate to marked erythematous mucosa with ulcerations and increased friability.

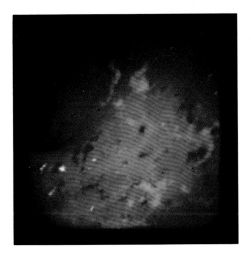 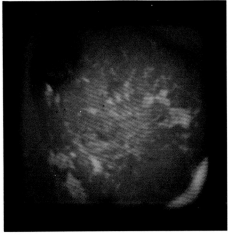

Fig. 91. A more advanced stage of active ulcerative colitis.

Fig. 92. Progressive ulcerative colitis with ulcerations, increased friability and a coarse, granular pattern.

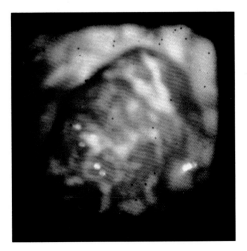

Fig. 93. Acute, active stage of ulcerative colitis. Markedly inflamed mucosa, coarse granular pattern and mucopurulent exudate.

height of the pseudopolyp, and as the fibrosis begins to involve long segments of colon, the walls become rigid and the lumen narrowed.

An additional use and indication for colonoscopy is the ability to allow biopsy in patients with longstanding disease strictures where questions of malignancy arise. The malignant potential is clear: as high as 2% per year after 10 years in some subsets of patients, with an overall incidence of cancer seven to 11 times higher than the normal population. Most cancers develop in the rectum and sigmoid; the next most common site is the transverse colon; and in 15%-20% of patients, multicentric or extensive malignancies develop. Morson has described the value of serial rectal biopsies in patients with chronic ulcerative colitis; some changes evident on biopsy precede the development of malignancy. Interpretative differences still remain, and the implications of these changes are still debated.

Granulomatous (Crohn's) Colitis

In contrast to chronic ulcerative colitis, which almost always involves the rectum, Crohn's disease (transmural colitis) has variable patterns of bowel involvement and clinical onset. It may involve any portion of the gastrointestinal tract. The terminal ileum and right colon often are involved, but total or segmental colonic involvement is also quite common. Less frequent are involvement of isolated segments of the proximal small bowel and involvement of the duodenum, stomach and esophagus, which usually accompany distal bowel disease.

The characteristic pathologic lesion involves all layers of the bowel wall (transmural), leading to inflammation, thickening, stenosis and linear ulcerations. Granulomas are found in half of patients, and enlarged or inflamed mesenteric lymph nodes also are common. Free perforation of the bowel is rare, but fistulas that develop between loops of bowel or other viscera are common. "Pseudopolyps" may develop but much less frequently than in patients with chronic ulcerative colitis.

Unlike chronic ulcerative colitis, which may be associated with mild perirectal disease, severe perirectal disease (abscess or fistulas) that heals poorly is not uncommon in patients with transmural colitis. Rectal bleeding usually occurs later than in chronic ulcerative colitis because the mucosa is secondarily involved and the disease may initially spare the rectum and rectosigmoid.

Colonoscopic findings are suggestive, subtle or characteristic. They may therefore be nonspecific and easily confused with those in chronic ulcerative colitis or other inflammatory diseases. If the rectum is initially free of disease, changes may not appear until the colonoscopist reaches higher in the colon.

My observations are that an early and subtle lesion in an apthous ulcer that is tiny, has a hemorrhagic center and is shallow (Fig. 94). This lesion occurs secondary to the submucosal lesion and produces a small mucosal slough. The surrounding mucosa is normal, as is the vascular pattern. Granulomas are occasionally found in such ulcers. As the submucosal disease progresses, longer segments of mucosa are lost due to either coalescence of the ulcers or submucosal undermining of mucosa. They may appear deep and linear and are characteristic when normal mucosa appears between such areas (Fig. 95).

Other findings include strictures, cobblestoning and mucosal bridging.

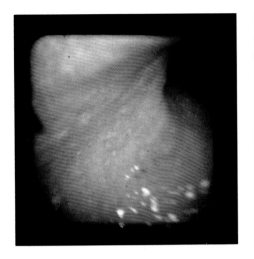

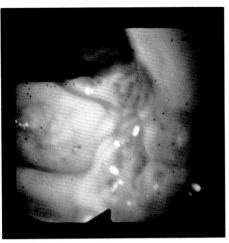

Fig. 94. Early stage of granulomatous colitis. Mucosa with apthous-appearing ulcers.

Fig. 95. Same patient as in Fig. 94. Development of longitudinal ulceration with normal-appearing, adjacent colonic mucosa.

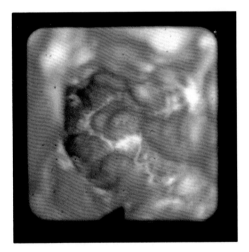

Fig. 96. Typical serpiginous ulcerations of granulomatous colitis.

With submucosal inflammatory disease, there is edema of the overlying mucosa, causing it to be elevated and bumpy; it thus acquires the appearance of a cobblestone road. When touched by biopsy forceps, it tends to be firmer than the mucosal elevations seen in inactive chronic ulcerative colitis, which is softer (Fig. 96).

As inflammatory injury repairs itself, fibrosis of the muscle wall develops, causing narrowing and strictures to develop. As in chronic ulcerative colitis, all inflammatory strictures require investigation and biopsy. Even though malignant tumors are less common in Crohn's disease, they do occur and must be excluded by colonoscopic examination and biopsy.

As the strictured area becomes larger, the colonic haustra are lost and the

lumen narrows. A pediatric endoscope (diameter, 0.7-1.0 cm) may be used to
pass the strictured area to allow examination of the right colon (Fig. 97).

Bridges of normal mucosa that connect ulcerated areas are more typical of
Crohn's disease than of chronic ulcerative colitis (see Fig. 101) but are seen in
both diseases.

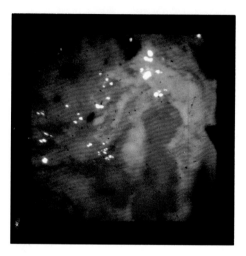

Fig. 97. *Large ulceration with colonic
stricture and fistula formation.*

Finally, severe perirectal disease, characteristic of transmural disease, is
detected by inspection and frequently the correct diagnosis can be made before
colonoscopy.

There are other important endoscopic features that must be kept in mind.
These features may be nonspecific, are seen in both forms of colitis and often
confuse the diagnostician. Examples are:

Strictures (Fig. 98)

Strictures may appear in Crohn's disease as fibrosis. They frequently develop
in both of these diseases. All inflammatory strictures must be investigated
thoroughly, both endoscopically and radiologically. Even though malignancy
is less common in Crohn's disease, it does occur and must be excluded. A
standard-size colonoscope may pass through the stricture. If such a colonoscope does not pass, a smaller instrument (pediatric type) should be used so
that the right side of the colon can be examined.

Narrowing and Shortening of the Colon
(Figs. 99a and 99b)

Diffuse narrowing of the colonic lumen and shortening of the bowel, with loss
of the normal colonic haustra, occur in Crohn's disease and chronic ulcerative
colitis.

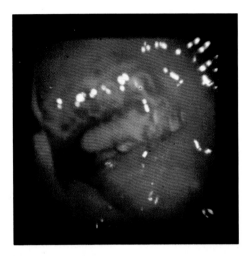

Fig. 98. Deep mucosal ulceration with luminal narrowing.

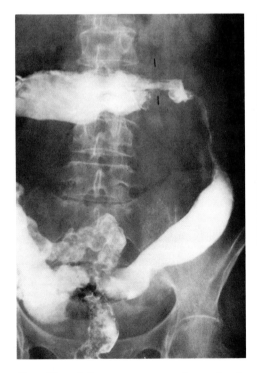

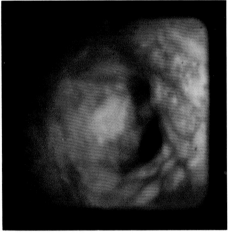

Fig. 99b. Endoscopic view of chronic ulcerative colitis with diffuse narrowing of the colonic lumen.

Fig. 99a. A barium enema view of substantial segmental narrowing and shortening of the colon. Loss of normal colonic haustrations is evident.

Pseudopolyps (inflammatory polyps)

These lesions are typically and more commonly associated with ulcerative colitis but occur in both diseases. They are long and fibular and may appear pedunculated. Although their appearance correlates with chronic illness, they may appear early in the disease (Figs. 100a and 100b). When the disease is severe, biopsy of these lesions documents the diagnosis because histologic examination reveals a characteristic lack of epithelium. When there are numerous lesions, biopsy is unnecessary. Pseudopolyps should be biopsied and removed if they are irregularly shaped, larger than 1 cm in diameter, friable or if their color is different from that of surrounding pseudopolyps. Because pseudopolyps have a tendency to bleed easily, snare-cautery polypectomy may be indicated.

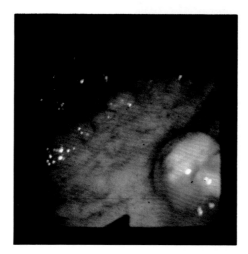 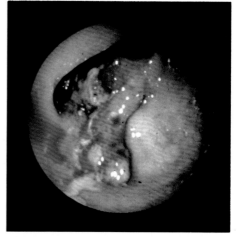

Fig. 100a. Inactive, atrophic mucosa with several scattered pseudopolyps.

Fig. 100b. Multilobulated, inflammatory polyp surrounded by chronically inflamed colonic mucosa.

Bridging

Mucosal bridges represent continuation of the mucosa and submucosa that are attached to the colonic wall. These structures may be seen in the healed stages of both ulcerative colitis and Crohn's disease (Fig. 101).

Skip Areas

This pattern is classic of Crohn's disease, in which areas of ulceration and disease are separated by segments of normal mucosa.

Cobblestoning

Regular bumpy elevations of the mucosa secondary to submucosal disease are characterized by a firmness that may be felt when biopsy forceps are applied.

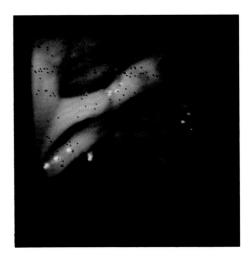

Fig. 101. *Mucosal bridging in the healing stage of ulcerative colitis.*

These structures are unlike the fine mucosal elevations seen in "burnt-out" ulcerative colitis, which are soft to the touch of the biopsy forceps.

Asymmetry

This feature is characteristic of Crohn's disease. Ulcerative colitis initially involves the colonic mucosa. However, on occasion, the inflammatory changes in a patient with severe ulcerative colitis may appear asymmetric. Biopsy may reveal an area of previous inflammation that has healed.

Ulceration

This feature is the major distinguishing characteristic of the two diseases. With progression of the submucosal disease, islands of mucosa are lost and sloughed, leaving large, long ulcers. In a few patients with severe chronic ulcerative colitis or dilatation of the colon, ulcerated mucosal areas may be seen as well. I have also seen active acute ulcerative colitis in association with longitudinal ulcerations. My impressions have been based on clinical correlations. Ulcers are seen histologically in association with inflammatory cells. Crohn's disease is accompanied by granulations. The overlap between diseases is less definite here.

MELANOSIS COLI

Melanosis coli (Fig. 102) is a curious, benign, reversible lesion characterized by mild to severe, dark brown to black pigmentation of the colonic and rectal mucosae. It occurs after prolonged use of anthracene-type laxatives, such as cascara and senna and may be accompanied by fecal stasis. When neoplastic

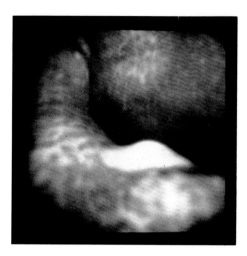

Fig. 102. *Marked melanosis coli shows dark brown mucosal pigmentation.*

polyps in the colon develop in patients with melanosis coli, they are pink to white and do not have the brown pigmentation of the mucosa. Therefore, it is not difficult to detect neoplastic polyps in the colorectum.

INFECTIOUS DISEASES

Acute infectious or parasitic colitis is rarely seen by colonoscopists because most diarrheal syndromes are diagnosed by other, more routine investigations. Endoscopic evaluation is usually the last diagnostic attempt.

It is sometimes difficult to differentiate acute infectious or parasitic colitis from more common inflammatory bowel diseases.

Colitis caused by specific parasites is usually seen in specific endemic areas. For example, acute amebic colitis is frequently difficult to differentiate from early ulcerative colitis. The characteristic features are new and old submucosal petechial hemorrhages and apthous ulcers similar to those seen in early Crohn's disease. In chronic amebic colitis, inflammatory changes and hemorrhagic, friable, edematous mucosa are most commonly seen in the cecal and rectosigmoid areas. Edematous mucosa and patchy, inflamed areas with petechial hemorrhages scattered in the colon and rectum are also common (Figs. 103-104).

The presence of amebic trophozoites or cysts can be demonstrated by appropriate amebic smears for diagnosis. Our method for obtaining specimens is as follows:

1. After colonscopic examination to the cecum, the instrument is withdrawn to the rectosigmoid area. The tip of the colonoscope is then slid gently along the colonic wall and withdrawn.

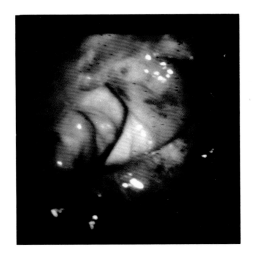 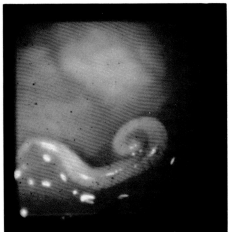

Fig. 103. Scattered submucosal hemor-   *Fig. 104.* Parasitic infestation of the
rhages in a patient with amebiasis.   cecum.

2. The tip is then immersed in a test tube that contains 5 ml of warm saline
   (37%C). After the specimens are obtained, they are stained with 5 ml of
   standard MIF solution (merthiolate, iodine, formalin).
3. The tube is centrifuged for a few minutes and then the supernatant partially spilled.
4. The remaining supernatant is swabbed, placed on a microscope slide and
   examined under an oil immersion lens. A search for the typical trophozoites
   or cysts is undertaken and should be successful if these organisms are
   present.

Of great interest is the finding of amebiasis in patients who require colonoscopic evaluation for other complaints, such as chronic abdominal pain and
change of bowel habits. In some such cases, the endoscopic picture may be
quite normal. Some minimal mucosal edema, prominent spasm or both may be
seen. Amebic trophozoites or cysts are sometimes found in fixed tissue biopsy
specimens obtained for other reasons. An unsuspected ameboma may be seen
as an ulcerated, friable, edematous tissue mass.

Schistosomiasis

Schistosomal colitis in the acute stage may resemble ulcerative colitis because
of the extremely friable mucosa. Biopsy specimens demonstrate an acute
polymorpholeukocytosis. In the chronic stage, mucosal nodes are seen and
consist of concentric fibrotic reactions around the granulomas (Fig. 105); inflammatory polyps are also noted.

Tuberculosis

The chronic lesion of tuberculous colitis, usually noted on the right side of the

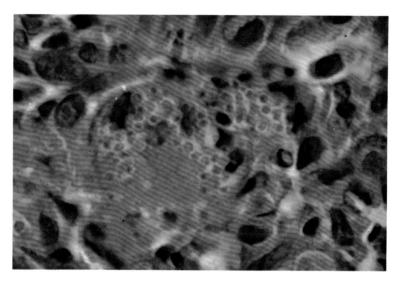

Fig. 105. Histologic features of schistosomiasis.

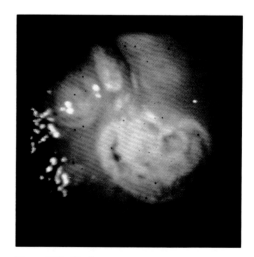

Fig. 106. Endoscopic view of colonic tuberculosis shows round or oval mucosal ulcerations in the right colon. This disease may be difficult to differentiate from Crohn's colitis.

colon, may be difficult to differentiate from that of granulomatous colitis. Tuberculosis may show extreme local alterations, with raised, edematous, granular, ulcerated lesions and markedly raised edges (Fig. 106). Tuberculous lesions may be diagnosed by endoscopic biopsy, which reveals acid-fast bacilli and caseating granulomas.

RADIATION COLITIS

Patients with radiation proctitis or colitis usually present with a constellation of symptoms that begin to appear a few months to several years after radiation therapy. The pelvis is the usual site of irradiation, and more than 4,000 rads are usually administered before any adverse effects are noted. Any segment of bowel within the irradiated area is subject to damage and ill effects manifested by early or late symptoms. Early symptoms are noted during treatment and consist of rectal bleeding and diarrhea, which indicate injury to the colonic mucosa. The colonoscopic picture may resemble that of acute colitis.

Late changes are usually stricture formation and occur anywhere in the bowel. Thus, there are many different colonoscopic findings (Figs. 107 and 108).

ISCHEMIC COLITIS

Ischemic colitis presents either spontaneously or as a complication of a surgical procedure on the abdominal aorta. The incidence after the latter ranges from 1% to 97%. In the spontaneous form, patients are usually elderly and have evidence of cardiovascular disease (cerebral vascular accident, myocardial infarction, cardiac valve disease, hypertension or peripheral vascular disease) and diabetes. The classic presentation of this disease is a sudden onset of excruciating colicky or steady abdominal pain, followed by bloody diarrhea. Abdominal

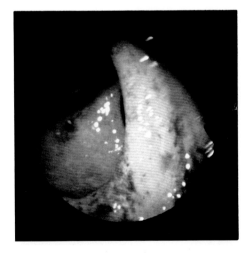

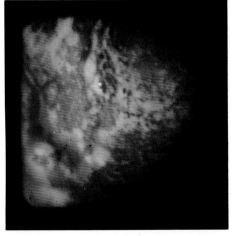

Fig. 107. Radiation colitis. Endoscopic view of the distal sigmoid colon shows fine, granular, friable and pale-appearing mucosa.

Fig. 108. Another endoscopic view of radiation colitis shows marked submucosal petechiae.

tenderness with or without rebound tenderness is localized over the affected segment of the colon. Patients may present with mild to moderate fever and leukocytosis, depending on the severity of the disease.

Endoscopic Characteristics

Because colonoscopic examination allows direct observation of the morphologic disease, it is useful in establishing the diagnosis. The disease is usually left-sided with a segmental distribution, and the rectum is usually spared. In mild to moderate cases, the affected segment of colonic mucosa is markedly edematous and hemorrhagic, with mucosal bulging and narrowing of the lumen (thumb printing on barium enema). The mucosal surface is frequently covered with purulent pseudomembranes, and/or mucosal erosions. In moderate to severe cases, there are more extensive changes, consisting of mucosal ulcerations and pseudomembranes with marked narrowing of the colonic lumen. Histologic evaluation of endoscopy biopsy specimens helps establish the diagnosis. The histologic diagnosis of ischemic colitis is highly suspected if hemosiderin deposits, necrosis, ulcerations or vascular thromboses are present (Figs. 109 and 110).

Course

Mild to moderate cases of ischemic colitis improve rapidly and endoscopy done serially over days to weeks shows no trace of stricture of the affected segment of colon. However, patients with acute disease should be considered medical emergencies; colonoscopy has no role in such patients—surgical intervention is frequently required.

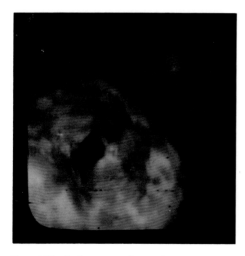
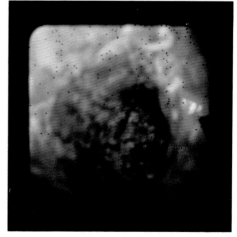

Fig. 109. *Ischemic colitis shows marked mucosal ulcerations and necrotic debris with luminal narrowing.*

Fig. 110. *Moderate to severe ischemic colitis with more extensive ulcerations, pseudomembranes, friability and a coarse, granular mucosa.*

PNEUMATOSIS CYSTOIDES INTESTINALIS

This rare disease entity usually presents as an intraluminal collection of gas bubbles within the colonic wall and mesentery. There are two forms, primary and secondary. The primary form is characterized by colonic involvement without associated disease, whereas in the secondary form, colonic involvement is associated with upper gastrointestinal pathology such as peptic ulcer, carcinoma of the stomach or, more commonly, chronic obstructive pulmonary disease.

Symptoms

The chief complaint is usually increasing constipation. Symptoms of diarrhea, flatulence, discomfort and bleeding are other presenting complaints.

Colonoscopic Characteristics

Clusters of cysts or globular masses are evident at endoscopy. They vary in size and project into the lumen in a scalloped manner. The overlying mucosa is somewhat pale, transparent and frequently hemorrhagic. Without any specific therapy, the condition may resolve spontaneously. Follow-up colonoscopic examinations at semiannual or annual intervals reveals that the large, cystlike structures have become smaller and more flattened (Figs. 111-115).

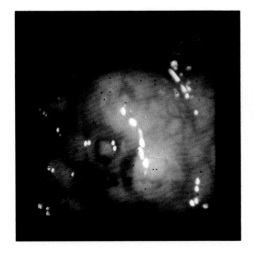 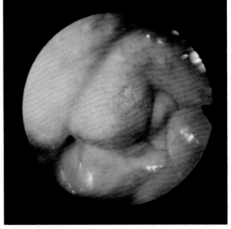

Fig. 111. Pneumatosis cystoides intestinalis. A solitary lesion is shown.

Fig. 112. Pneumatosis cystoides intestinalis. Several air-filled, submucosal, cystic structures are evident.

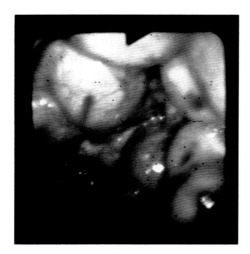 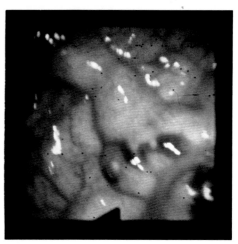

Fig. 113. Clusters of cysts in pneumatosis cystoides intestinalis with submucosal hemorrhage. The patient presented with increasing constipation and guaiac-positive stools.

Fig. 114. Resolving phase of pneumatosis cystoides intestinalis. Less prominent cystic structures with residual submucosal hemorrhage are evident.

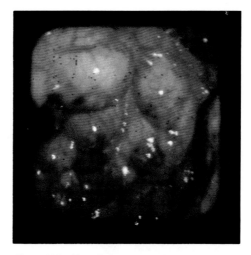

Fig. 115. Another case of pneumatosis cystoides intestinalis with cobblestone-like mucosa that must be differentiated from inflammatory bowel disease.

Therapy

The only approach is to wait to see if the disease resolves spontaneously. Surgical procedures are reserved for complications (bleeding, perforation, or obstruction).

Breathing high concentrations of oxygen for several days has led to complete resorption of such cysts.

ANGIODYSPLASTIC LESIONS

There are several types of vascular lesions of the colon. Examples are venectasis or varicose veins, cavernous hemangiomas, capillary hemangiomas and angiomas or telangiectasias. Because of the difficulty of differentiating these lesions, they are classified as angiodysplasias (Figs. 116-118).

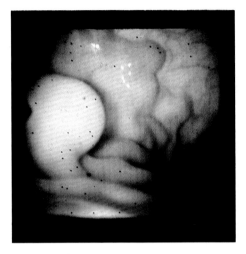

Fig. 116. Varicose veins of the colon. A polypoid-appearing varix is seen in the sigmoid colon.

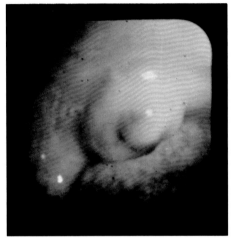

Fig. 117. Solitary angiofibroma of the sigmoid colon. The patient presented with repeated episodes of rectal bleeding.

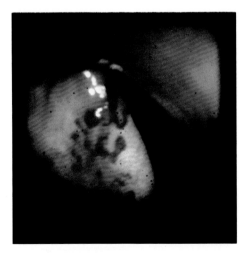

Fig. 118. Telangiectatic lesion of the cecum.

That these lesions are sources of lower gastrointestinal bleeding has become apparent since the advent of angiography and colonoscopy. They are difficult to recognize either intraoperatively or pathologically. Although they may be present in any area of the colon, they typically occur in the right side of the colon and cecum, usually in patients over 65 years of age. They are usually less than 0.5 cm in diameter and may be solitary or multiple. They usually are not associated with angiodysplasias of the skin or other organs. As noted, they may be detected angiographically, especially if the patient is bleeding actively. However, they may be recognized endoscopically as intramucosal or submucosal lesions. They appear as oval, round or stellate flecks that are usually friable when touched.

Since biopsy can cause hemorrhage, and fulguration, especially in the cecum, and may lead to perforation, biopsy and fulguration usually are not done. If such a lesion is noted to be bleeding actively, resection of the colon usually is advised or pharmacoangiography is done (Figs. 119-121).

COLONIC ENDOMETRIOSIS

Endometriosis involving the colon is not frequently recognized because the diagnosis is difficult. Of the 8%-15% of women with endometriosis, 3%-34% have bowel involvement.

Endometriosis predominates in premenopausal women (age range, 25 to 46 years), usually those who are multiparous or who have late pregnancies.

Endometrial implants usually involve the sigmoid colon. Crampy lower abdominal pain, episodic bloody stools, alternating constipation and diarrhea, and small stools are the consequences of endometrial implants. Bowel symptoms are usually, but not necessarily, cyclic and frequently related to menstrual periods.

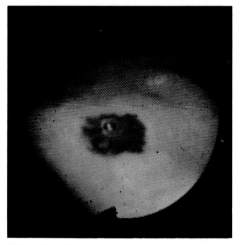

Fig. 119. Vascular ectasia of the cecum.

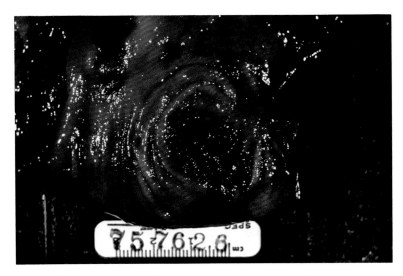

Fig. 120. *Same case as in Fig. 119. Operative specimen shows vascular ectasia after injection of indigo carmine.*

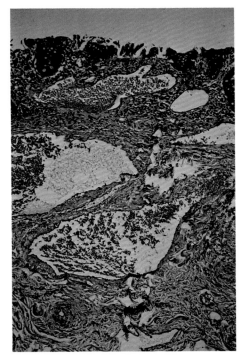

Fig. 121. *Histologic section of vascular ectatic lesions.*

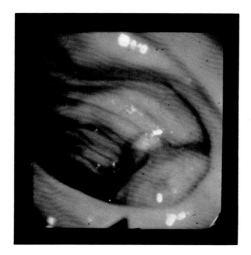 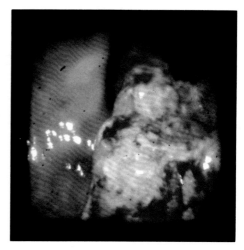

Fig. 122. Endometrioma of the sigmoid colon. Area of mucosal irregularity and granulation. Biopsy confirmed the diagnosis.

Fig. 123. Polypoid endometrioma of the sigmoid colon resembling an inflammatory polyp.

Endoscopic Appearance

Establishing the diagnosis is more difficult. Endoscopy may prove inconclusive. Most commonly, a partially obstructing extrinsic mass is found. Occasionally, marked tenderness is encountered. Endoscopic biopsy does not obtain tissue from the deep layers and usually does not prove the diagnosis. Endometrial tissues rarely are seen in the bowel mucosa (Figs. 122 and 123).

Pathology

The findings at surgery correlate with the constellation of symptoms and with the findings of barium enema. Patients without gastrointestinal complaints but with endometriosis found at surgery usually have involvement of the colonic serosa. In contrast, patients with gastrointestinal symptoms usually have deeper involvement of the bowel wall and may require colotomy to excise the lesion. The mucosa usually adheres to the submucosa, but mucosal involvement is uncommon. Patients previously treated with hormones frequently have lesions that ulcerate the mucosa. Because frozen sections can accurately determine if the disease is endometriosis, such studies should be done in all young and middle-aged women who are at increased risk so that resection of the colon can be avoided (Fig. 124).

PEUTZ-JEGHERS SYNDROME

In 1921, Peutz described a syndrome of polyposis of the small intestine associated with pigmented lesions of the skin. In 1949, Jeghers described polyposis

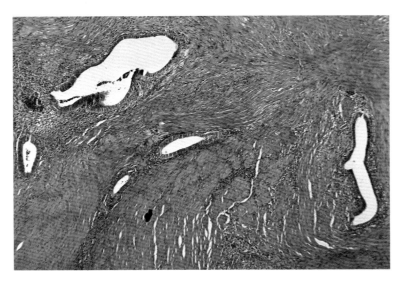

Fig. 124. *Histologic section of endometriosis of the colon.*

of the intestinal tract with mucocutaneous pigmentation. In 1954, Bruwer named this condition Peutz-Jeghers syndrome, which in the classic description consists of mucocutaneous melanin pigmentation, intestinal polyposis and a family history of the disease.

From 45% to 50% of children of affected parents are either partially (with pigmentation only) or totally (with pigmentation and polyposis) affected. The syndrome is probably inherited through an autosomal dominant gene. Half of all reported cases have had no familial involvement; these cases may represent a defect in a mendelian-dominant gene of the patient.

The clinical onset is usually before age 30 and is characterized by recurrent, severe, colicky abdominal pain. Rectal bleeding or melena is not uncommon. Hematemesis may be seen with gastric or duodenal polyps. Many patients have been anemic. Because of the large size of some polyps, intussusception or bowel obstruction is not unusual.

The polyps occur throughout the gastrointestinal tract but are most commonly seen in the jejunum and ileum, followed in frequency by the colon, rectum, stomach, duodenum and appendix. A rare case of esophageal polyposis as the presenting feature of Peutz-Jeghers syndrome has also been described.

Endoscopic Appearance

The appearance and size of these polyps vary, but they resemble adenomatous polyps. They may be sessile or pedunculated. One or more polyps are sometimes noted, but these structures usually present as numerous nodules in the intestinal mucosa. Micropolyposis within the bowel wall has been demonstrated in this entity (Figs. 125-128).

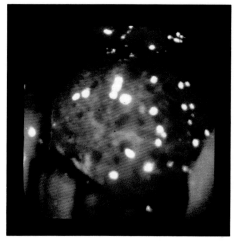

Fig. 125. Hamartomatous polyp in Peutz-Jeghers syndrome.

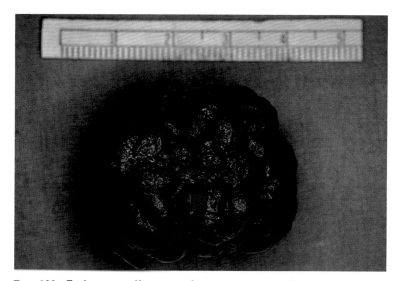

Fig. 126. Endoscopically excised specimen (same as in Fig. 125).

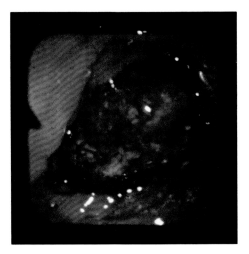

Fig. 127. *Hamartomatous lesion resembling adenomatous polyp.*

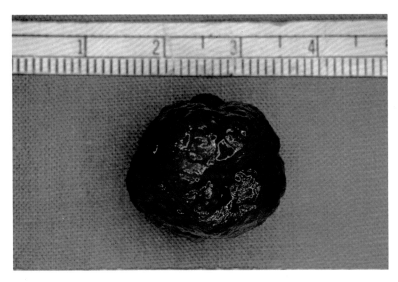

Fig. 128. Excised specimen (same as in Fig. 127).

Histology

Histologic examination of the polyps reveals that most are hamartomas, which are abnormal rearrangements of normal tissue. These lesions are composed of columnar absorptive cells, Paneth cells and goblet cells. All the cellular elements are well differentiated from the point of origin of the polyp. A tree branch arrangement of the fibromuscular stroma, which arises from smooth muscle within the muscularis mucosa, characterizes such polyps (Figs. 129 and 130). Because the mucosal malformation may be situated deep within the muscularis mucosa, care must be taken not to confuse this entity with malignant invasion. Such misinterpretations are likely because numerous mitotic figures are typical of hamartomas. These lesions are benign and have a much lower malignant potential than do adenomatous polyps.

Differential Diagnosis

Peutz-Jeghers syndrome must be differentiated from familial polyposis, which rarely involves the small intestine and is a highly premalignant condition, from Gardner's syndrome, which is also highly premalignant but in which there are few polyps scattered throughout the gastrointestinal tract and is associated with soft tissue tumors and osteomas, from juvenile polyposis, which is characterized by multiple polyps in young patients, and is not premalignant and commonly affects the rectum, and from adenomatous polyps of the colon and rectum, which have a malignant potential.

There are several other clinical features of Peutz-Jeghers syndrome. Even though young women have this syndrome, 5% of 180 cases reported in women

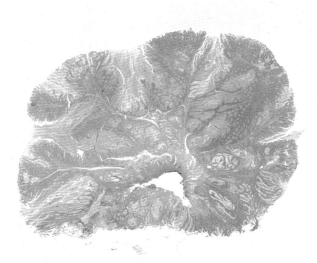

Fig. 129. Typical histologic appearance of a hamartomatous polyp.

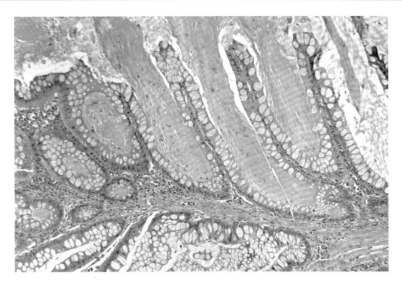

Fig. 130. Closeup histologic view of a hamartomatous polyp.

up to 1966 had associated ovarian tumors or cysts (an especially remarkable finding since many of the patients were young women). Bladder and nasal polyps have also been occasionally reported in such patients. More rarely, bronchial polyps, external exostoses and clubbing of fingers have been associated findings.

The question of malignancy infrequently arises in Peutz-Jeghers syndrome. Although gastrointestinal malignancies have been reported at a slightly higher frequency than would be expected on the basis of chance, the distribution of such tumors is in accord with that of the general population, and such tumors are not restricted to geographic locations where hamartomas are prevalent. Furthermore, adenomatous colonic, stomach and small bowel polyps have been found to be malignant in such patients. Coexisting adenomatous polyps have a premalignant potential, but hamartomatous polyps do not.

Treatment

Treatment of this syndrome is difficult. Because of the diffuse distribution and intermittent growth patterns of the polyp, a definitive prophylactic approach is not possible.

Endoscopy and polypectomy is a relatively conservative approach for polyps that can be reached (those in the stomach, duodenum, terminal ileum, colon and rectum). Annual or biannual examinations after polypectomy can help keep these areas free of polyps and can reduce the likelihood of malignant degeneration since these accessible areas are where malignant tumors are likely to develop. However, recurrent intussusception, hemorrhage or anemia may necessitate surgical intervention after accurate localization.

JUVENILE POLYPS AND JUVENILE POLYPOSIS

Juvenile polyps are hamartomas, not adenomatous polyps. These lesions may appear in adults, although they more often occur in young persons.

These polyps are pedunculated and have a smooth surface (Figs. 131-133). They are sometimes sessile. On histologic section, they typically show mucus-

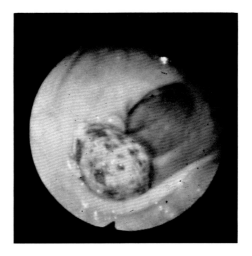

Fig. 131. *Juvenile polyp of the sigmoid colon.*

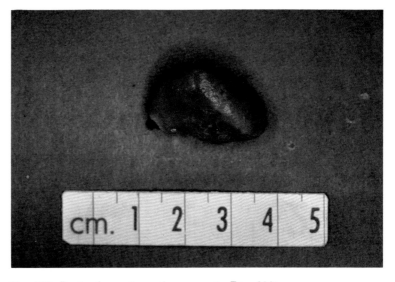

Fig. 132. *Excised specimen (same as in Fig. 131).*

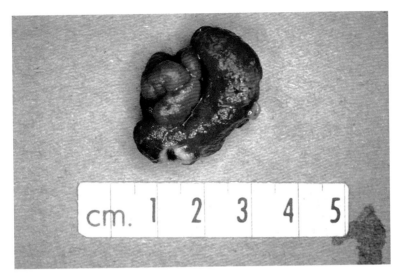

Fig. 133. Another excised juvenile polyp. The head of this type of polyp is frequently deformed and covered by a thick mucoid material.

filled cystic spaces, with an increased mucosal stroma and branching of the glands (Fig. 134). In addition, numerous capillaries are seen.

These polyps rarely, if ever, undergo malignant degeneration. The usual complication of such polyps in the colon is bleeding. Most undergo spontaneous degeneration and usually slough.

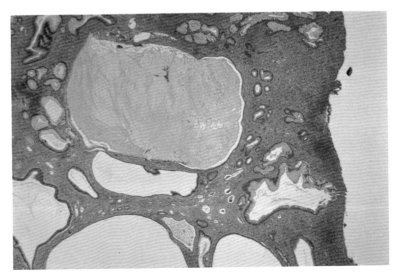

Fig. 134. Histologic appearance of a juvenile polyp shows mucus-filled cystic spaces.

Juvenile polyps usually are found in the rectum and left colon and are rarely seen in the right colon. They are more common in boys than girls.

Since some such lesions bleed, it may be necessary to excise them endoscopically. Some patients complain of abdominal pain because of intussusception, and these polyps occasionally prolapse through the anus.

In some instances, numerous juvenile polyps are found scattered throughout the entire colon (Fig. 135). Such cases do not require immediate surgical intervention. An alternative plan is to do frequent colonoscopic polypectomy. Any polyps deemed suspicious should be excised for histologic evaluation (Fig. 136).

The following case serves as an illustration of the management of juvenile polyposis.

A 7-year-old female presented to us with a strong family history of colonic polyposis and colon cancer. At the age of 6 this child reportedly had intermittent bloody bowel movements. A barium enema was performed at that time and revealed multiple colonic polyps. Subsequent colonoscopy confirmed the finding of multiple colonic polyposis. Several polyps were excised and pathology revealed juvenile polyposis. A total colectomy was advised by the child's physician. We saw the child because the family was reluctant to have her undergo this type of extensive surgery. We performed a total colonoscopy and found numerous polyps ranging in size from 0.3-1.5 cm. scattered throughout the entire colon. We removed approximately 80 of the larger polyps from the

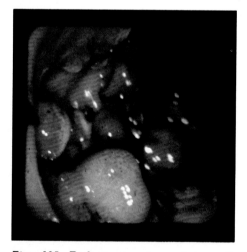

Fig. 135. Endoscopic view of juvenile polyposis in a 15 year-old girl. The patient had a subtotal colectomy at age 11. Since that time, she has undergone several endoscopic polypectomies. Altogether, approximately 250 polyps were excised colonoscopically from the rectum and sigmoid colon.

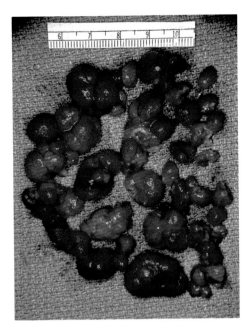

Fig. 136. Numerous excised specimens in a patient with juvenile polyposis (same as in Fig. 135).

left and right colon at two sessions. Pathology revealed all of these lesions to represent juvenile polyps. We have not recommended that this child have any surgical intervention at this time.

Some physicians feel that the natural history of this entity is that of spontaneous degeneration once the child reaches adolescence. However, others believe that these polyps may change toward the adenomatous types with their attendant risks. This has rarely been reported, and whether these adenomas arise de novo or are a degeneration of juvenile polyps is open to conjecture.

We feel that patients with juvenile polyposis should have the larger lesions excised and examined histologically. If no adenomatous changes are found, these patients can be followed at bi-annual or annual intervals with no need for surgical intervention unless neoplastic changes are demonstrated.

We have had one patient without family history of colonic neoplasm, who had a subtotal colectomy with ileosigmoidostomy for juvenile polyposis. We subsequently removed more than 250 polyps in several sittings from the remaining colon and rectum. These polyps markedly diminished due to repeated resection and/or spontaneous degeneration when the patient reached adolescence. During the course of resection over several years, none of these polyps was found to be adenomatous.

In conclusion, each patient with juvenile polyposis should be individually treated, either endoscopically or surgically, depending upon family history, age, general condition and pathology.

HAMARTOMAS

As described above, these lesions are similar to juvenile and Peutz-Jeghers polyps. They are smooth and are associated with numerous mucus-filled cysts having an abundant stroma that contains smooth muscle fibers and capillaries. When these lesions are small (less than 1.0 cm), it is difficult to distinguish between inflammatory, juvenile and Peutz-Jeghers polyps.

HYPERPLASTIC OR METAPLASTIC POLYPS

Hyperplastic or metaplastic polyps are found in 20%-30% of all excised colonic polyps. In addition, as many as 90% of all lesions less than 3 mm in diameter were found to be hyperplastic. Most authors agree, after extensive histologic studies, that this type of non-neoplastic polyp never undergoes malignant degeneration.

These polyps are most frequently found during routine colonoscopic examinations for other problems. They usually are an incidental finding of little consequence. They are removed only if there is uncertainty as to whether they are adenomatous polyps. Removal is usually accomplished with a biopsy forceps (Fig. 137).

They appear endoscopically as minute elevations, slightly paler than the surrounding colonic mucosa. In addition, their surface has a glistening appearance (Fig. 138).

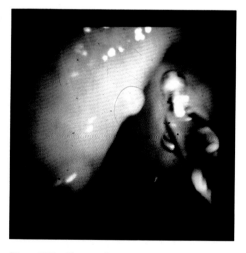

Fig. 137. Hyperplastic polyp measuring approximately 0.3 cm. Biopsy forceps in view.

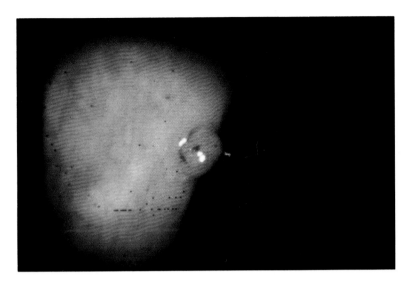

Fig. 138. Hyperplastic polyp resembling an adenomatous lesion.

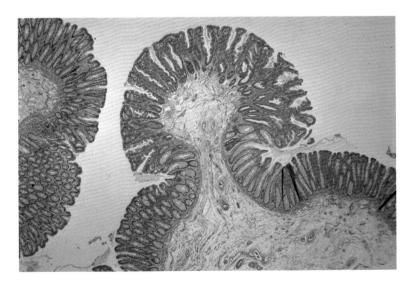

Fig. 139. Histologic appearance of a hyperplastic polyp.

Histologic studies show that these polyps have a normal glandular distribution. Cell numbers are somewhat increased, and the epithelium demonstrates a mild papillary character (Fig. 139).

SUBMUCOSAL TUMORS

Lipomas

Lipomas are the most common benign, non-neoplastic, submucosal tumors found in the colon and rectum. They are most frequently located in the colon, usually on the right side. They are uncommon in the rectum.

When a patient presents with symptoms (usually obstructive from intussusception) the lipoma is large (more than 4-5 cm in diameter).

Endoscopic Appearance

Lipomas vary in size from a few millimeters to several centimeters. They are mostly sessile, smooth, nonlobulated and slightly yellow (Fig. 140). If they are small and soft, it may be difficult to visualize them through the colonoscope. Since they are covered with colonic mucosa, their shape may change, and they thus may be confused with or lost in redundant colonic mucosa. The surface of lipomas often becomes erythematous and hemorrhagic, especially those that are pedunculated or polypoid. The overlying mucosa may also become necrotic and ulcerated and may bleed (Figs. 141 and 142).

If the lesion is firm, other submucosal polypoid tumors such as leiomyomas, leiomyosarcomas, neurofibromas and granular cell myoblastomas, should be considered.

When the lesion is pushed with the biopsy forceps or the tip of the colonoscope, the surface indents much like that of a soft cushion. This response is usually referred to as a "cushion sign."

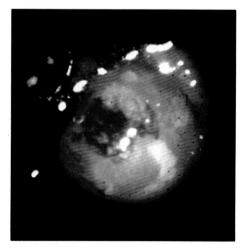

Fig. 140. Lipomatous lesion of the cecum with a hemorrhagic surface.

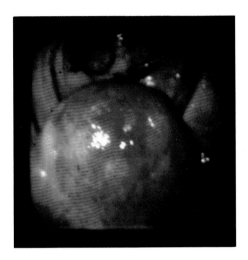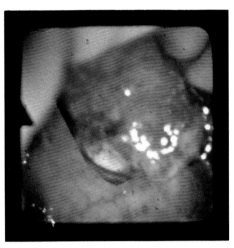

Fig. 141. Lipoma with markedly erythematous, overlying mucosa.

Fig. 142. Large, firm lipoma with overlying mucosal ulceration.

Treatment

Lipomas have relatively little clinical importance. They are frequently found by
chance during colonoscopy.

When a lipoma is large, soft and yellow, the endoscopic diagnosis is easily
made. If the colonoscopic examination reveals the lesion to be a typical lipoma,
I believe it should not be excised unless it is less than 1.5 cm in diameter, has a
pedicle or has a narrow base. Snare-wire transection of a lipoma may not only
be difficult but may also perforate the bowel. Perforation sometimes occurs
because the submucosal nature of this lesion requires a longer transection time,
which may allow the cautery burn to extend through the colon wall. An asymptomatic lesion can be restudied endoscopically on an annual basis or every
two years to insure that they are not getting larger.

If symptoms are related to the lesion or if the lipoma is large, firm and ulcerated, excision is advised, usually by laparotomy (Figs. 143 and 144). Intussusception is common in symptomatic lesions.

Lymphoid Polyps (Benign Lymphoma,
Lymphoid Hyperplasia and
Lymphocytoma)

Lymphoid polyps are most commonly found in the rectum (especially in the
distal portion) and rectosigmoid area. They vary in size and are usually not
larger than 1 cm. Some may even be as small as a pinpoint. They are usually
white, sharply circumscribed and flat. When larger than 1.0 cm in diameter,
they tend to form a sessile or pedunculated polypoid elevation (Fig. 145). These

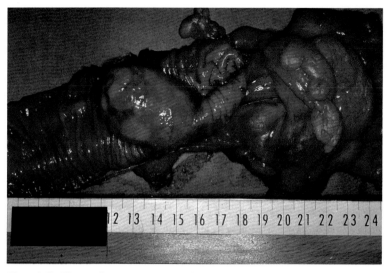

Fig. 143. Excised operative specimen of ulcerated lipoma arising from the ileocecal valve.

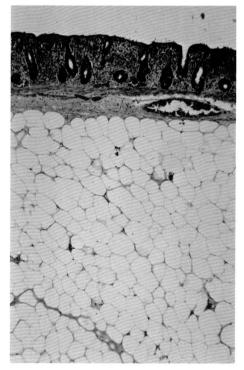

Fig. 144. Histologic appearance of a lipoma.

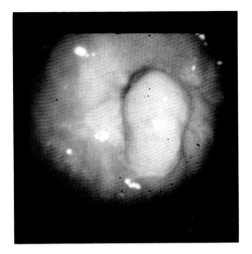

Fig. 145. *Benign lymphoid polyp of the rectum. The lesion was covered by a normal colonic mucosa.*

elevations may be mistaken, endoscopically, for neoplastic or carcinoid polyps. Often, multiple lymphoid polyps, of a similar size, are present.

If the lesion is polypoid, particularly when it is located in the rectum, up to 10 cm from the anal verge, it may be excised colonoscopically using the snare-wire and cautery unit.

Leiomyomas

Leiomyomas (Fig. 146) are smooth muscle tumors of the colon and rectum. We have removed five such lesions colonoscopically; four were located in the colon

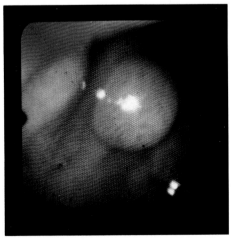

Fig. 146. *Endoscopic view of leiomyoma of the right colon.*

and one in the rectum. They were small, ranging in diameter from 0.8 to 1.3 cm, and grossly appeared to be adenomatous lesions (Fig. 147). Pathologic examination revealed that they were leiomyomas. The four colonic lesions were pedunculated, and the rectal lesion was sessile. Although these lesions are submucosal or intramural, they can be confused with neoplastic polyps (Fig. 148).

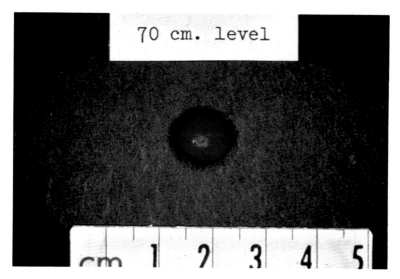

Fig. 147. *Excised specimen (same as in Fig. 146).*

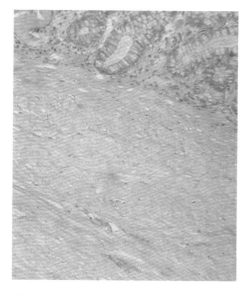

Fig. 148. *Histologic appearance of a leiomyoma of the colon.*

Treatment

When these lesions are pedunculated, they may be excised locally by transecting the stalk with a snare-wire. If they are sessile and situated in the colon, colonoscopic excision is contraindicated.

Carcinoid Tumors

Carcinoid tumors have been found throughout the gastrointestinal tract from the cardia of the stomach to the anorectal junction. These tumors arise from the enterochromaffin cells (Kulchitsky) in the crypts of Lieberkuhn. The appendix is the most common site of carcinoid tumors.

Carcinoids of the colon are most commonly found in the rectum. These lesions grow slowly and have a low potential for malignancy. They are usually asymptomatic and are incidental findings at colonoscopy. The carcinoid syndrome rarely occurs with rectal carcinoids.

Endoscopically, carcinoid tumors typically appear as round, tan lesions situated in the submucosa (Figs. 149 and 150). Usually, they are less than 1 cm in diameter. If they are this size and lie below the peritoneal reflection, they may be excised endoscopically. Lesions of this size usually are benign. Because of their submucosal location, endoscopic excision is dangerous above the peritoneal reflection.

Increased resistance is felt during endoscopic transection of this tumor or other submucosal lesions (leiomyoma or lymphoma) because of their location. Large lesions (more than 2 cm in diameter) usually are invasive and require operative resection (Figs. 151-153).

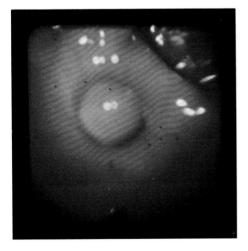

Fig. 149. Carcinoid tumor of the rectum.

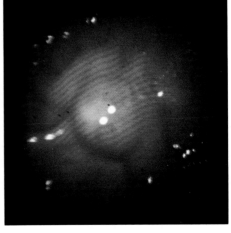

Fig. 150. Carcinoid tumor of the rectosigmoid.

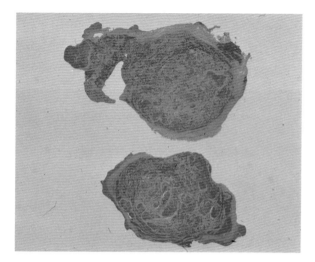

Fig. 151. Histologic appearance of a rectal carcinoid tumor (excised endoscopically).

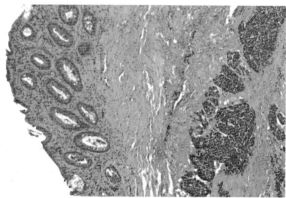

Fig. 152. High-power view of a carcinoid tumor excised endoscopically.

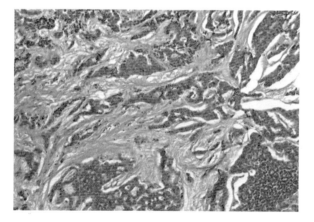

Fig. 153. High-power view of the histologic features of a carcinoid tumor.

Granular-Cell Myoblastoma

Granular-cell myoblastoma is a rare submucosal tumor of the gastrointestinal tract found from the oral cavity to the rectum. Extraintestinal lesions have been demonstrated in other organs, including the respiratory tract, thyroid gland and biliary tree. Histologically, they were thought to have arisen from the myoblast, the precursor cell of striated muscle. Some investigators, using electron microscopy, have recently demonstrated neural elements in such tumors, implying a relation between neural tumors and granular-cell myoblastoma. Because of difficulty in establishing the exact origin of such tumors, they have been classified as tumors of "unsettled origin." They are neoplastic.

Histologic studies show that these cells have a polygonal shape, with a characteristic highly granular cytoplasm.

Endoscopically, they resemble other submucosal tumors, such as carcinoids, lymphomas and leiomyomas. They usually are covered by normal mucosa, and deep biopsy may confirm the true nature of the lesion (Figs. 154 and 155).

If the tumors are less than 1 cm in diameter and are situated in the rectum within the 10 cm level, they may be excised endoscopically for a definitive diagnosis. Lesions larger than 1 cm in diameter, which usually are ulcerated, should be excised surgically (Figs. 156-158).

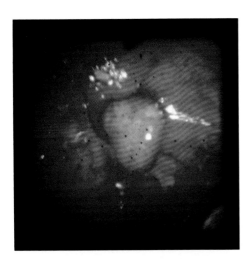

Fig. 154. Granular-cell myoblastoma of the cecum.

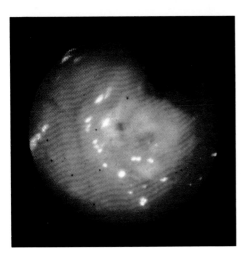

Fig. 155. Ulcerating granular-cell myoblastoma of the cecum.

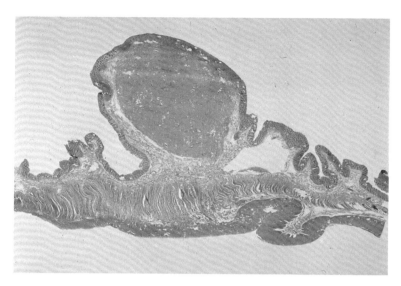

Fig. 156. Low-power view of the histologic features of a granular-cell myoblastoma.

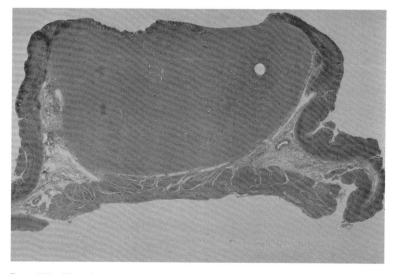

Fig. 157. Histologic appearance of an ulcerated granular-cell myoblastoma.

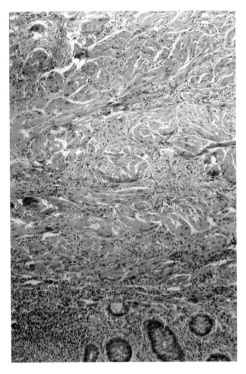

Fig. 158. High-power view of a granular-cell myoblastoma.

11

Neoplastic Polypoid Lesions

CLASSIFICATION OF ADENOMAS

Polyps (the Greek word for "little feet") are the most common neoplasms of the colon. Numerous classifications have evolved based on morphologic, gross or histologic appearances. Of the neoplastic adenomatous polyps, papillary and villous lesions predominate. Although these terms refer only to gross characteristics of the polyps, a more precise descriptive classification based on histologic patterns is available and will be referred to in this chapter. This classification includes tubular adenomas, villotubular adenomas and villous adenomas.

Tubular Adenomas

If more than 75% of the polyp contains tubular elements it is classified as a tubular adenoma. These tumors may be sessile or pedunculated. If pedunculated, the head is spherical and smooth, but in large pedunculated or sessile polyps, the head may be lobulated. The pedicle of a pedunculated polyp consists of stroma, blood vessels and lymphatics. It is formed by the pull of peristalsis on the mucosa and submucosa. Long stalks occur more commonly in the sigmoid, descending and transverse colon. Peristaltic contractions are more forceful in the sigmoid and decline proximally.

Villotubular Adenomas

These have also been known as villoglandular or mixed polyps. They are more common than was previously recognized. Both villous and tubular architectures are found within these polyps. If the mixture consists of more than 25% of either tubular or villous elements, the polyp is a villotubular adenoma. This type of polyp is frequently multilobulated and has a malignant potential. The incidence of invasive cancer in villotubular adenomas in our studies was 8.2%, and the incidence of carcinoma in situ was 13.4%.

124

Villous Adenomas

These tumors are the least common neoplastic polyps. They are often sessile and vary greatly in size and shape. If more than 75% of the polyp consists of villous elements, it is classified as a villous adenoma. These polyps have the highest incidence of malignant change.

Because they are frequently larger and sessile, villous adenomas often have to be removed in piecemeal fashion via the colonoscope. On occasion, they involve more than half the circumference of the colorectal wall. Although their coloring may sometimes be similar to that of adjacent normal mucosa, the colonoscope helps determine the exact margins of such lesions.

Histologic Criteria

Histologic grading of malignant colonic adenomas is based on structural or cytologic changes. Structural changes refer to shape and topographic features of the neoplastic glands, whereas cytologic changes refer to individual neoplastic cells. Generally, both methods of grading concur. An exception is well-differentiated infiltrating adenocarcinomas, which often contain abundant mucus. In these cases, structurally evident carcinomas appear cytologically benign. Thus, structural grading supercedes when the two classifications disagree. In other words, histologic diagnosis of carcinoma in adenomas depends not on the appearance of the neoplastic cells but on the gross architecture of the adenomas.

Carcinoma and Grading of Dysplasia

In polyps, dysplastic changes are often found. They may be mild, moderate or severe. At times, this finding is of little practical importance. It certainly is less important than whether a polyp is malignant or benign, and we place less emphasis on degree of dysplasia than on the presence or absence of malignancy.

Invasion

Malignant invasive changes in colonic adenomas imply "crossing of the muscularis mucosa" (not "crossing the basement zone"). Therefore, in invasive carcinoma, malignant cells penetrate through or beneath (or both) the layer of the muscularis mucosa.

Superficial carcinoma is defined as a lesion in which carcinomatous cells involve the superficial fibers of the muscularis mucosa but do not invade the muscularis mucosa (intramucosal carcinoma). Although true cancers, these lesions are not malignant in a clinical sense and do not metastasize. However, once the muscularis mucosa is penetrated, they behave as infiltrating cancers.

When reporting the histologic appearance of an excised polyp, one must distinguish between superficial and invasive carcinoma since this distinction has important implications regarding management. When cancer cells penetrate the muscularis mucosa, this change must be regarded as invasive carcinoma. This statement applies to both sessile and pedunculated polyps. To determine the presence and degree of penetration or invasion, the polyp must be excised completely, and multiple fixed tissue sections with proper orientation must be prepared.

ADENOMAS

Morphologic Features, Anatomic Distribution and Cancer Potential

In our hands, after 11 years of experience, colonoscopy allows detection of malignant and premalignant lesions of the colon at an early stage. Only the future will tell whether it is accompanied by a high cure rate and whether it prevents the development of cancer of the colon.

The most far-reaching contribution of colonoscopy will prove to be the ability to identify and remove premalignant or early malignant lesions. When polypoid lesions of the colon are diagnosed by barium enema or colonoscopy, they should be totally excised and evaluated histologically. The procedure of choice in approaching colorectal polyps has been the technique of snare-cautery resection via the colonoscope, which we introduced in 1969. This technique has proven reliable, safe and accurate. We have excised colonoscopically more than 7,800 colonic polyps larger than 0.5 cm in diameter, with negligible morbidity and no mortality during the past 11 years. This success is dependent on many factors, including technical skill and, I believe most importantly, judgmental decisions that determine which polyp should be removed.

In reviewing the histopathologic characteristics of a polyp, one should distinguish between superficial and invasive cancer.

Although there is general agreement concerning the malignant potential of adenomas of the colon, areas of controversy persist, particularly with respect to the potential and frequency of cancer development. The concept of a polyp-cancer sequence hinges on an accurate analysis of abnormal changes in colon adenomas and of the frequency with which these changes occur. Also of interest is how these alterations explain why polyps develop in different regions of the

Table 6. Colonoscopic Polypectomy: Histologic Findings for 7,015 Neoplastic Polyps (Sep. 1969–Dec. 1979)

	Number	Percent
Benign	5,130	73
Dysplasia	625	9
Carcinoma in situ	850	12
"Malignant polyps"	410	6
Adenomas with invasive cancer	337	5
Polypoid cancer	73	1
Total	7,015	100

colon. Histologic findings for 7,015 neoplastic polyps, which we excised colonoscopically are shown in Table 6.

Previous reports describing these relations have been based on lesions removed either at surgery or via rectosigmoidoscopy from the distal colorectum. With the advent of colonoscopy, a new era has been entered. It is now possible to examine systematically the entire colon of large numbers of persons with symptomatic and asymptomatic lesions at various stages of development.

Tubular Adenomas, or Adenomatous Polyps

If more than 75% of the polyp contains tubular elements, it is called a tubular adenoma (Figs. 159-171).

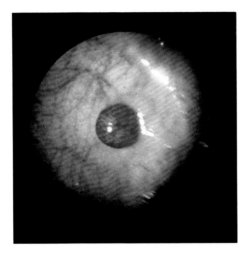

Fig. 159. Sessile tubular measuring 0.8 cm in diameter.

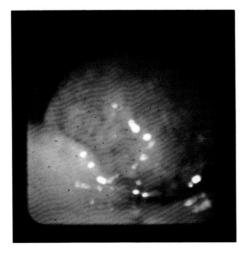

Fig. 160. Narrow-based, sessile tubular adenoma measuring 1.5 cm in diameter.

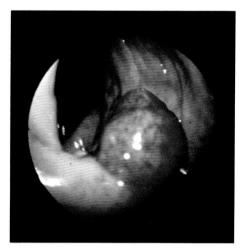 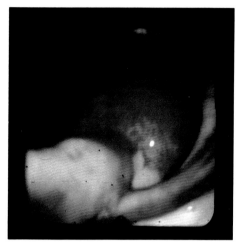

Fig. 161. *Pedunculated tubular adenoma measuring approximately 1.3 cm in diameter.*

Fig. 162. *Pedunculated tubular adenoma on a long stalk measuring 1.5 cm in diameter.*

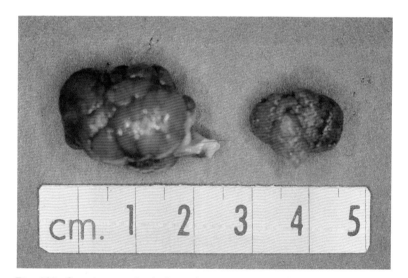

Fig. 163. *Specimens of tubular adenomas resected colonoscopically.*

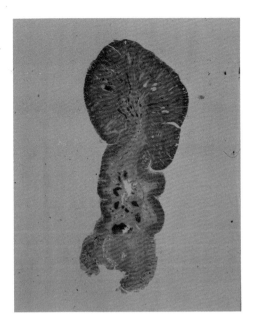

Fig. 164. Histologic appearance of a tubular adenoma with a head and long stalk.

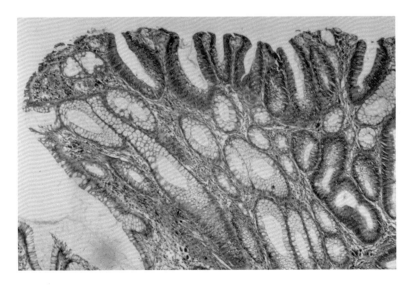

Fig. 165. Histologic appearance of a tubular adenoma and normal mucosa.

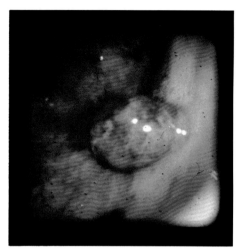 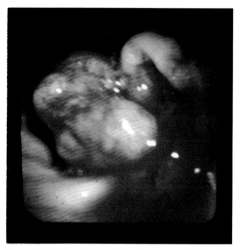

Fig. 166. Endoscopic view of a sessile tubular adenoma measuring 1.2 cm in diameter. Microscopic examination showed marked dysplasia in the adenoma.

Fig. 167. Pedunculated, somewhat friable polyp in the sigmoid measuring 1.7 cm in diameter. The excised specimen showed numerous focal areas of carcinoma in situ in a tubular adenoma.

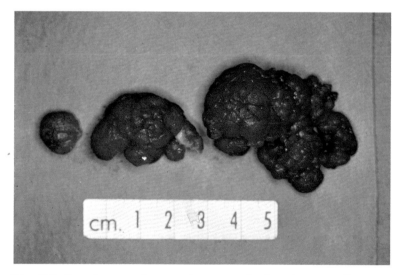

Fig. 168. Two large polyp specimens excised endoscopically contained carcinoma in situ.

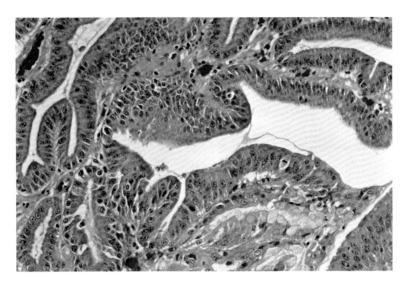

Fig. 169. Histologic appearance of a tubular adenoma showing dysplasia.

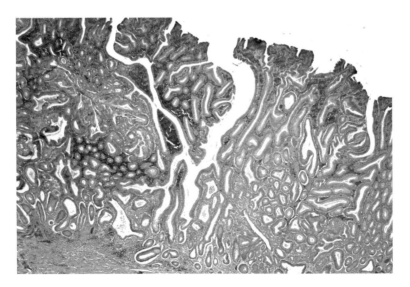

Fig. 170. Histologic appearance of a tubular adenoma containing carcinoma in situ.

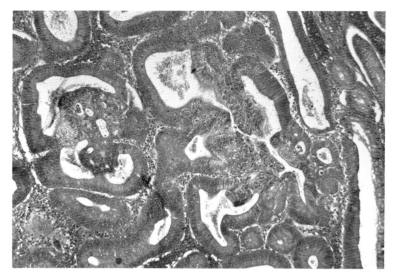

Fig. 171. *High-power view of a tubular adenoma containing carcinoma in situ.*

Villotubular Adenomas, or Villoglandular or Mixed Polyps

These tumors are more common than has been previously recognized. Both villous and tubular architectures are found. If the mixture consists of more than 25% of either tubular or villous elements, the polyp is called a villotubular adenoma (Figs. 172-185).

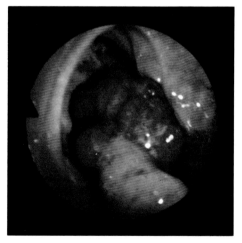

Fig. 172. *Pedunculated, lobulated villotubular adenoma measuring approximately 1.5 cm in diameter.*

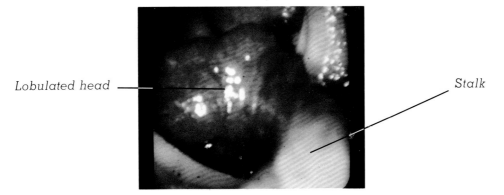

Lobulated head ———   ——— Stalk

Fig. 173. *Endoscopic view of a peduncu-lated, lobulated villotubular adenoma measuring approximately 2.0 cm in diameter.*

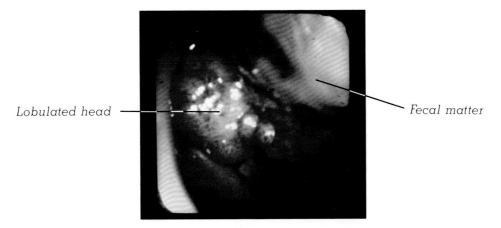

Lobulated head ———   ——— Fecal matter

Fig. 174. *Multilobulated, sessile polyp measuring 4.0 cm in diameter, partially covered with mucus.*

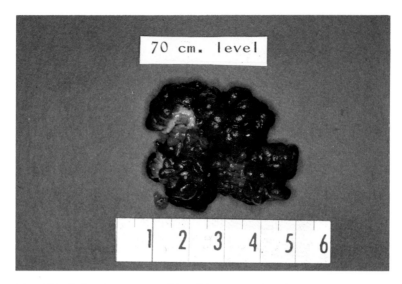

Fig. 175. Polyp (same as in Fig. 174) excised endoscopically in four sessions.

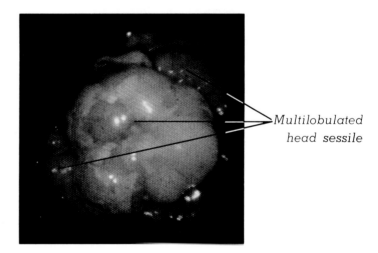

Multilobulated
head sessile

Fig. 176. Endoscopic view of a lobulated, villotubular adenoma measuring 3.0 cm in diameter.

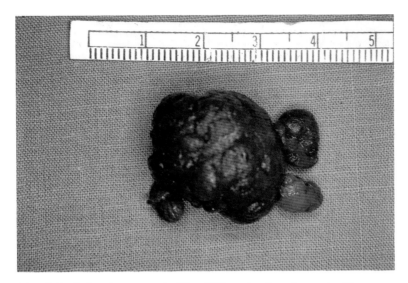

Fig. 177. Polyp (same as in Fig. 176) excised endoscopically.

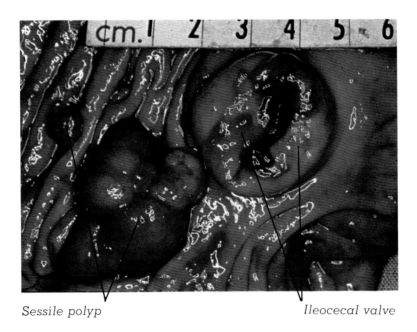

Sessile polyp   Ileocecal valve

Fig. 178. Right colon resected surgically shows a large sessile polyp (containing carcinoma in situ) adjacent to the ileocecal valve.

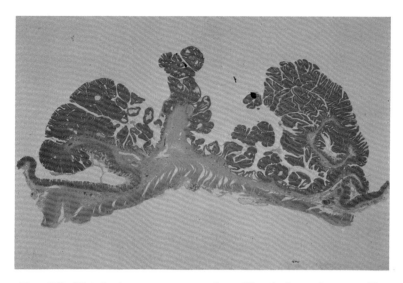

Fig. 179. Histologic appearance of a villotubular adenoma (Note marked lobulation) resected surgically.

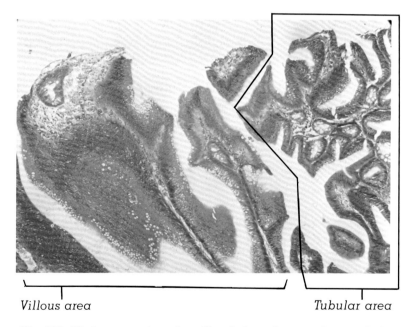

Villous area   Tubular area

Fig. 180. High-power view of a villotubular adenoma shows tubular and villous elements.

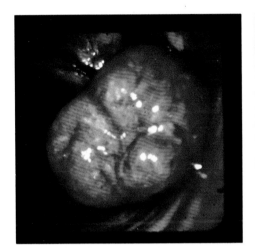 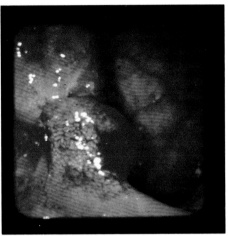

Fig. 181. Endoscopic view of a villotubular adenoma with a concave surface. The
histology revealed extensive carcinoma
in situ.

Fig. 182. Endoscopic view of a wide-
based, somewhat friable, sessile villotubular adenoma.

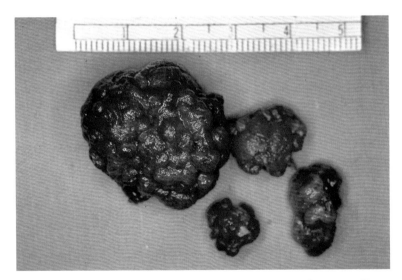

Fig. 183. Polyp (same as in Fig. 182) excised endoscopically in
several segments.

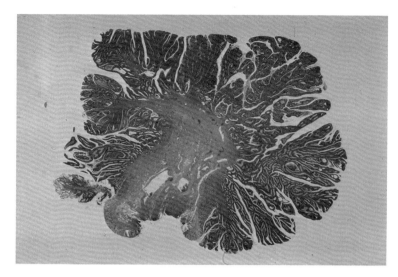

Fig. 184. *Low-power view of one segment of the same polyp shown in Fig. 182.*

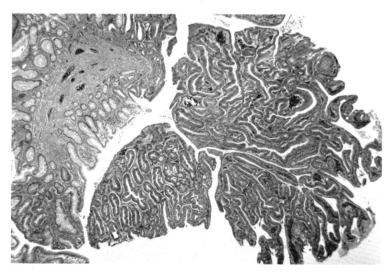

Fig. 185. *Histologic appearance of the polyp shown in Fig. 182 include an area of carcinoma in situ.*

Villous Adenomas

These lesions are the least common form of neoplastic polyp. They are often sessile and may vary greatly in size and shape. In our classification, if more than 75% of the polyp consists of villous elements, it is classified as a villous adenoma. These tumors have the highest tendency toward malignant degeneration (Figs. 186-197).

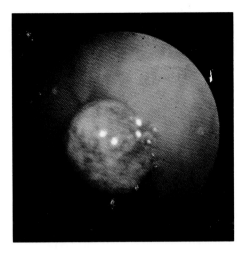

Fig. 186. Sessile villous adenoma in the sigmoid colon measuring approximately 1 cm in diameter.

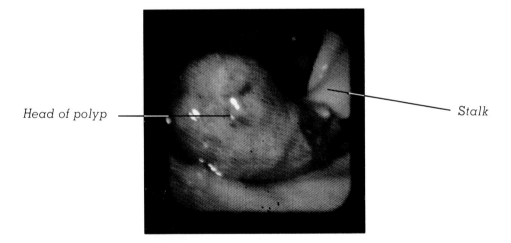

Fig. 187. Pedunculated villous adenoma measuring approximately 2.5 cm in diameter.

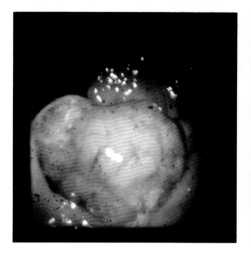 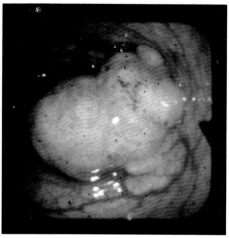

Fig. 188. Sessile villous adenoma measuring approximately 2.0 cm in diameter.

Fig. 189. Large (approximately 4 cm in diameter), wide-based sessile villous adenoma.

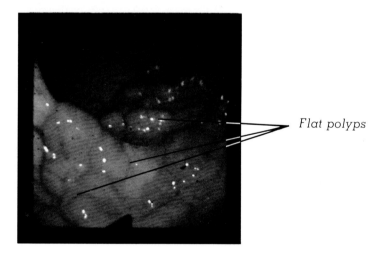

Flat polyps

Fig. 190. Flat villous adenoma ("creeping moss" appearance).

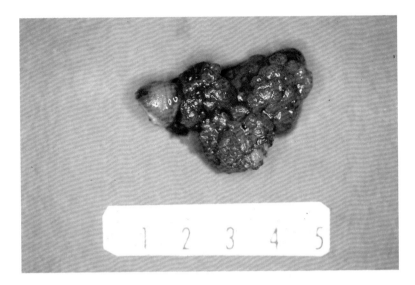

Fig. 191. Pedunculated villous adenoma resected endoscopically in three segments.

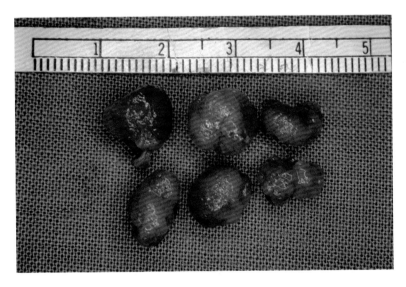

Fig. 192. Sessile polyp excised endoscopically in six segments (see Fig. 189).

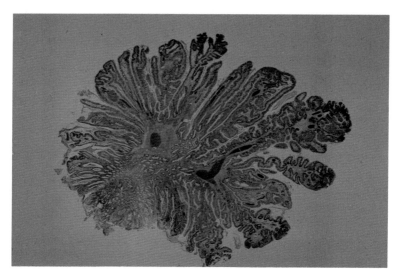

Fig. 193. Histologic appearance of a sessile villous adenoma excised completely in one segment (see Fig. 186).

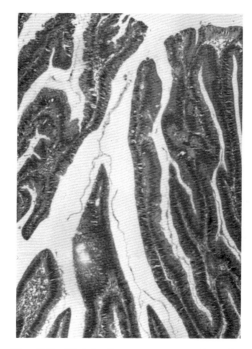

Fig. 194. Histologic appearance of a villous adenoma.

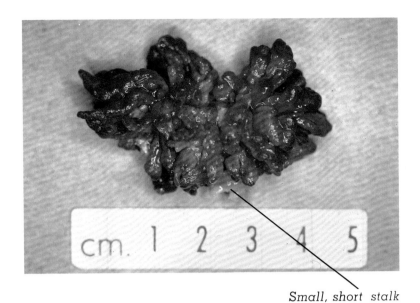

Small, short stalk

Fig. 195. Large villous adenoma on a small, short stalk.

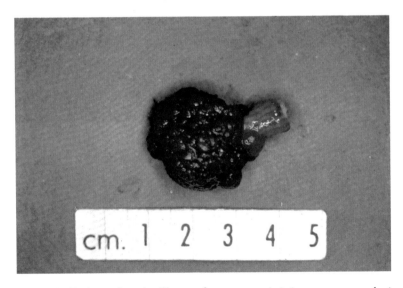

Fig. 196. Pedunculated villous adenoma containing numerous foci of carcinoma in situ.

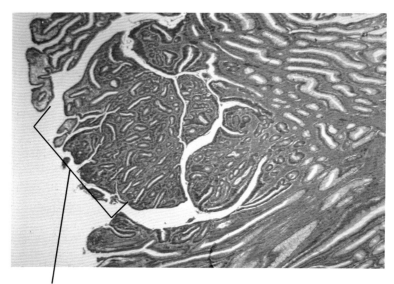

Carcinoma in situ

Fig. 197. *Histologic appearance of a villous adenoma containing foci of carcinoma in situ (see Fig. 196).*

Distribution of Adenomas in Regions of the Large Bowel

The types and locations of polyps are shown in Table 7. This table shows the distribution of adenomas in various regions of the colon for each of the three categories mentioned. Most adenomas are in the sigmoid colon, followed by the descending colon. But, in all zones, the highest percentage of adenomas is tubular, followed by villotubular and villous (Table 7).

Table 7. Distribution of Types of Adenomas in the Large Bowel

Region of large bowel	Tubular		Villotubular		Villous	
	Number	Percent	Number	Percent	Number	Percent
Rectum	228	5	113	6	77	14
Sigmoid	2,199	48	801	44	199	36
Descending colon	1,022	22	441	24	138	25
Transverse colon	572	13	210	12	42	7
Right colon	549	12	252	14	99	18
Total	4,570	100	1,817	100	555	100

The graphic presentation also illustrates the fact that the sigmoid has the highest frequency of tubular, villotubular and villous lesions, followed by the descending colon. The percentage of villous adenomas is higher in the rectum and the right colon than in other regions (Fig. 198).

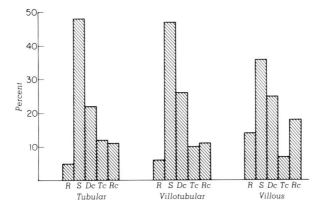

Fig. 198. *Distribution of types of adenomas in the large bowel. R, rectum; S, sigmoid; Dc, descending colon; Tc, transverse colon; Rc, right colon.*

Distribution of Pathologic States of Adenomas in Each Region of the Large Bowel (Table 8)

In each region, the highest percentage of lesions is benign. Less frequently, dysplasia, carcinoma in situ and invasive carcinoma are present. The table also shows that dysplasia, carcinoma in situ and invasive carcinoma are most common in the sigmoid colon, followed by the descending colon.

These differences are illustrated graphically in Fig. 199. The highest frequency of each lesion is in the sigmoid colon. It is also evident that the fre-

Table 8. Distribution of Pathologic Stages of Adenomas in Each Region of the Large Intestine

Region of large bowel	Total number	Benign*	Dysplasia*	Carcinoma in situ*	Invasive carcinoma*
Rectum	418	297(6)	31(5)	66(8)	24(7)
Sigmoid	3,199	2,221(43)	295(47)	481(57)	202(60)
Descending colon	1,601	1,266(25)	115(18)	170(20)	50(15)
Transverse colon	824	632(12)	99(16)	63(7)	30(9)
Right colon	900	714(14)	85(14)	70(8)	31(9)
Total	6,942	5,130(100)	625(100)	850(100)	337(100)

* Numbers followed by percentages in parentheses.

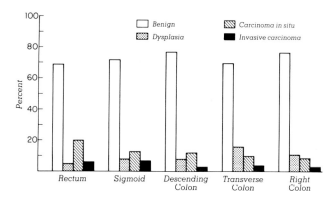

Fig. 199. *Distribution of pathologic stages of adenomas in each region of the large bowel.*

quency of invasive carcinomas is higher in the sigmoid than is dysplasia or carcinoma in situ. This difference is statistically significant at the 5% level.

Relative Frequencies of Pathologic Stages of Adenomas

Most (60%-78%) tubular, villotubular and villous adenomas are benign. A higher percentage of villous than tubular or villotubular lesions have dysplasia, carcinoma in situ and invasive carcinoma (Table 9).

Table 9. Relative Frequencies of Pathologic Stages in Adenomas

Adenomas	Benign*	Dysplasia*	Carcinoma in situ*	Invasive carcinoma	Total*
Tubular	3,559(78)	362(8)	520(11)	129(3)	4,570(100)
Villotubular	1,238(68)	185(11)	240(13)	154(8)	1,817(100)
Villous	333(60)	78(14)	90(16)	54(10)	555(100)
Total	5,130	625	850	337	6,942

* Numbers followed by percentages in parentheses.

Size of Adenomas in Association with Carcinoma in Situ

With increasing size of adenomatous polyps (tubular, villotubular and villous), the frequency of carcinoma in situ increases, with the highest frequency occurring in large villous adenomas (Table 10).

This observation is shown graphically in Fig. 200, where the increased incidence of carcinoma in situ corresponds to the size of the polyp. It is greater in the villous adenomas than in the other lesions.

Table 10. Size of Adenoma Related to Carcinoma in Situ (CIS)

Size of adenoma (cm)	Tubular		Villotubular		Villous	
	Number	CIS (%)	Number	CIS (%)	Number	CIS (%)
0.5-0.9	1,858	82(4.5)	157	7(4.5)	42	3(7.1)
1.0-1.9	2,100	298(14)	898	77(8.6)	260	22(8.5)
2.0-2.9	499	108(22)	556	94(17.0)	106	17(16)
3.0 + − 2	113	32(28)	206	62(30.0)	147	48(33)
Total	4,570	520(11.4)	1,817	240(13.2)	555	90(16.2)

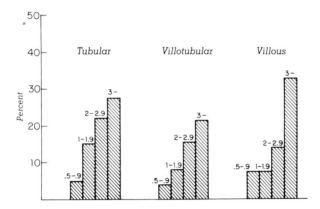

Fig. 200. Size of adenoma (in centimeters) in association with carcinoma in situ.

Size of Adenomas in Association with Invasive Carcinoma

Similarly, the frequency of invasive carcinoma increases with the increasing size of adenomas, again with the highest frequency occurring in villous adenomas. Although there is also an increased incidence of malignant degeneration with increasing size, it is of interest that invasive carcinoma can and does occur in small polyps (Table 11).

Table 11. Size of Adenoma Related to Invasive Carcinoma (IA)

Size of adenoma (cm)	Tubular		Villotubular		Villous	
	Number	IA (%)	Number	IA (%)	Number	IA (%)
0.5-0.9	1,858	6(0.3)	157	4(2.5)	42	1(2.4)
1.0-1.9	2,100	75(3.6)	898	63(7.0)	260	14(5.4)
2.0-2.9	499	34(6.8)	556	60(10.8)	106	18(17.0)
3.0 +	113	14(12.4)	206	27(13.1)	147	21(14.3)
Total	4,570	129(2.8)	1,817	154(8.5)	555	54(9.7)

This observation is shown graphically in Fig. 201. Some of the largest villous or villotubular adenomas require surgical removal rather than endoscopic excision. The sharper increase in the incidence of invasive carcinoma in the villous and the villotubular adenomas compared to the tubular variety is also seen.

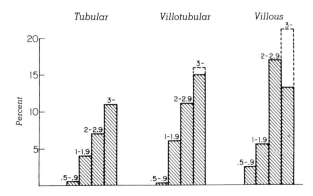

Fig. 201. *Size of adenoma (in centimeters) in association with invasive carcinoma.*

Correlation of Total Number of Adenomas and Carcinoma in Situ

A very high correlation is present; the correlation of significance is 98% as the number of adenomas per patient increases, the incidence of carcinoma in situ also increases (Fig. 202).

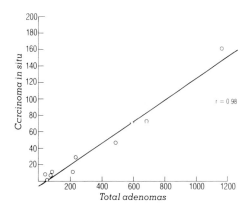

Fig. 202. *Regression comparison of total adenomas and carcinoma in situ.*

Correlation of Total Number of Adenomas and Invasive Carcinoma

This correlation is also very high, 97%. As the number of adenomas per patient increases, the number of invasive carcinomas increases (Fig. 203).

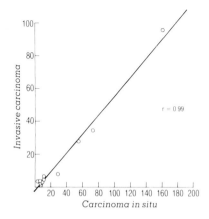

Fig. 203. *Regression comparison of carcinoma in situ and invasive carcinoma.*

Correlation of Carcinoma in Situ and Invasive Carcinoma

This correlation is also very high (99%.) The incidence of carcinoma in situ and of invasive carcinoma increase together (Fig. 204).

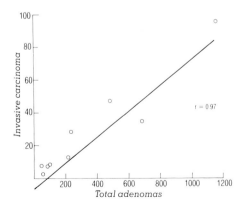

Fig. 204. *Regression comparison of total adenomas and invasive carcinoma.*

Endoscopic Appearance of Adenomas with Invasive Carcinoma and Polypoid Carcinoma

The successful management of patients with polyps that contain invasive carcinoma or polypoid carcinoma depends largely on the careful selection of the lesion and patients. There are several characteristic features of invasive carcinoma and polypoid cancer that, in most cases, make them recognizable endoscopically. These endoscopic and gross features are as follows:

Deformity of the Head of the Polyp

This change occurs when a major portion of the adenomatous polyp contains invasive cancer, while the benign portion of the polyp retains its smooth, regular features (Figs. 205-208).

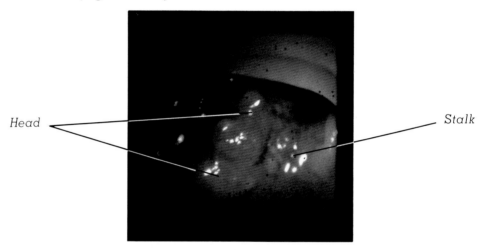

Head   *Stalk*

Fig. 205. *Endoscopic view of a pedunculated polyp with an irregular and ulcerated head (containing invasive carcinoma).*

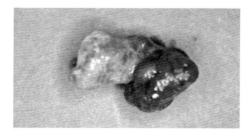

Fig. 206. *Pedunculated polyp excised endoscopically showing a markedly deformed head (containing invasive carcinoma).*

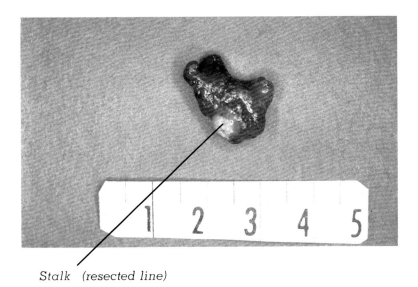

Stalk (resected line)

Fig. 207. *Polyp excised endoscopically showing a markedly deformed head. The histologic features included invasive carcinoma close to the line of resection.*

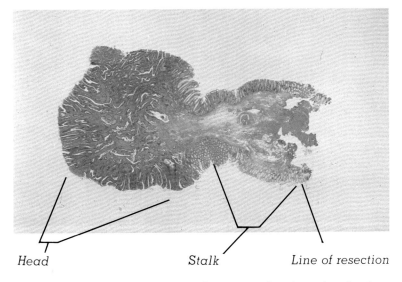

Head   Stalk   Line of resection

Fig. 208. *Histologic appearance of an excised pedunculated polyp. Almost the entire head is replaced by carcinoma. The stalk and line of resection are not involved.*

Deep Ulceration

In wide-based, sessile polyps or discoid-shaped polyps that show deep ulceration, this finding indicates advanced cancer, and the polyps should not be excised endoscopically. However, pedunculated polyps that show ulceration are amenable to endoscopic resection (Figs. 209-211).

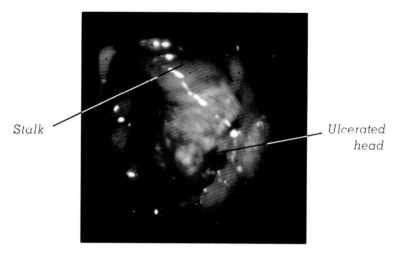

Stalk   *Ulcerated head*

Fig. 209. *Endoscopic view of a penduculated polyp with a deep ulceration of the head.*

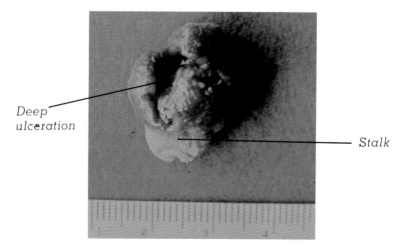

Deep ulceration   *Stalk*

Fig. 210. *An excised specimen of the same polyp contains invasive carcinoma (see Fig. 209).*

Invasive carcinoma

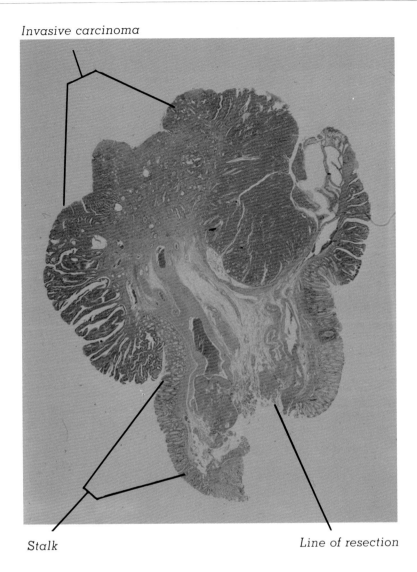

Stalk   *Line of resection*

Fig. 211. *Histologic appearance of the same polyp containing invasive carcinoma (see Figs. 209 and 210).*

Concave Surface, with Irregular Nodular Appearance

This finding is seen most commonly in pedunculated polyps with invasive cancer. If the stalk appears short and wide, the polyp can be resected endoscopically in a piecemeal fashion. If this change is seen in wide-based, sessile polyps, partial excision is recommended for histologic evaluation (Figs. 212 and 213).

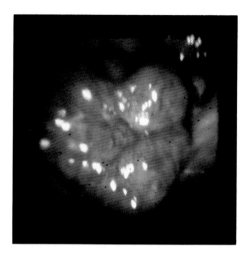

Fig. 212. Endoscopic view of a polyp having a concave surface.

Carcinoma

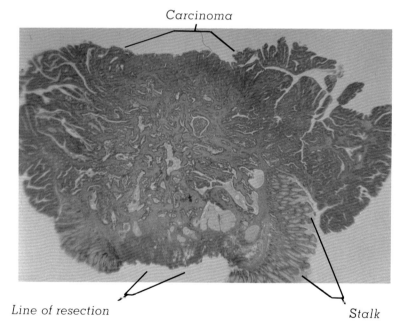

Line of resection   Stalk

Fig. 213. Histologic appearance of the same polyp containing invasive carcinoma (see Fig. 212). The line of resection is involved.

Granular, Friable Surface

This change is seen in pedunculated and sessile polyps that contain invasive cancer or are polypoid carcinomas. It is sometimes seen without deformity, concavity or deep ulceration of the polyp. This change implies that the cancer is not deeply invasive. The operator usually sees this feature in small sessile lesions (Figs. 214-217). Even small polyps with deeply invasive cancer become deeply ulcerated.

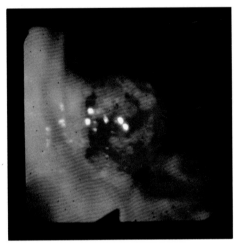

Fig. 214a. *Endoscopic view of a sessile polyp measuring approximately 1.0 cm in diameter and having a granular, friable surface.*

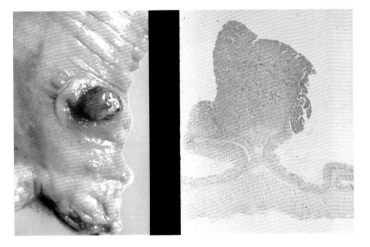

Fig. 214b. *A 42-year-old female with rectal bleeding underwent colonoscopic examination. In the sigmoid colon a polypoid lesion with a granular, friable surface was noted (operative specimen left). Biopsy revealed evidence of invasive carcinoma, and the patient underwent sigmoid resection (photomicrograph right).*

Carcinoma   Carcinoma

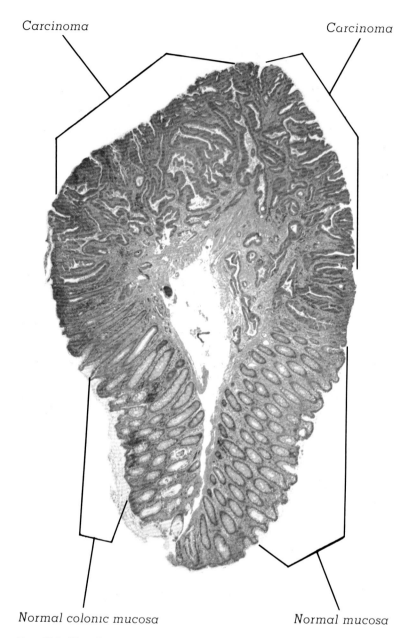

Normal colonic mucosa   Normal mucosa

Fig. 215. *Histologic appearance of an excised specimen containing invasive carcinoma (see Fig. 214).*

If the operator touches the polyp with the tip of the biopsy forceps or instrument and it moves easily and freely from the colonic wall, superficial invasion is likely. If the polyp and colonic wall move together, there is invasion beyond the submucosa. After lassoing the polyp, and tenting the lesion, the entire

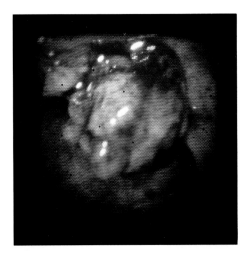

Fig. 216. Endoscopic view of a sessile polypoid lesion containing invasive carcinoma.

Invasive carcinoma

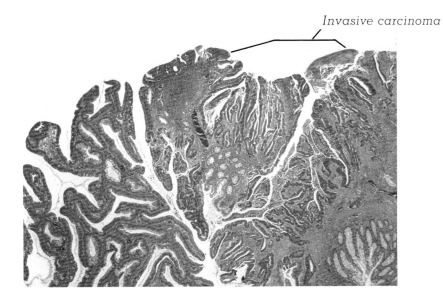

Fig. 217. Histologic appearance of the same polyp containing invasive carcinoma (see Fig. 216).

colonic wall is tented as well, thus implying that invasion through the submucosa has taken place. In such cases, the polyp should not be excised from its base, unless the lesion is located 10 cm below the peritoneal reflection in the rectum and has a considerably narrow base.

Discoloration

This finding indicates any localized uneven change in the usual color of the adenoma. The discoloration may be a white area in the polyp. Deformity or irregularity of the surface may or may not be present (Figs. 218 and 219).

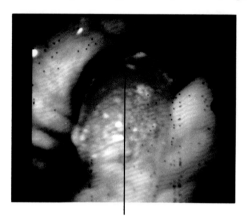

Discolored areas

Fig. 218. *Endoscopic view of a pedunculated polyp with discolored areas in the head. Numerous foci of invasive carcinoma were seen in the discolored zones.*

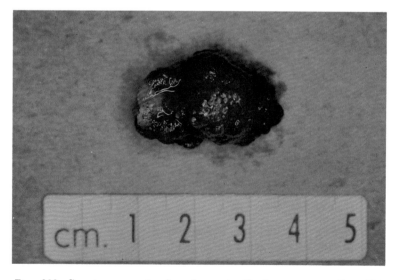

Fig. 219. *Specimen excised endoscopically (same as in Fig. 218). Several areas of invasive carcinoma were seen in the whitish-appearing part of the head.*

Disproportion in Size Between the Head and the Stalk

In such cases, the head is small in comparison to the size and length of the stalk. In this type of polyp, superficial cancer or low-grade invasive change is common. In our opinion, this is due to the slow growth of the malignant process in which the head has the tendency to slough (Figs. 220-222).

If, while transecting the head or stalk of the polyp, the operator experiences markedly increased resistance to transection, this implies that carcinomatous tissue is being divided.

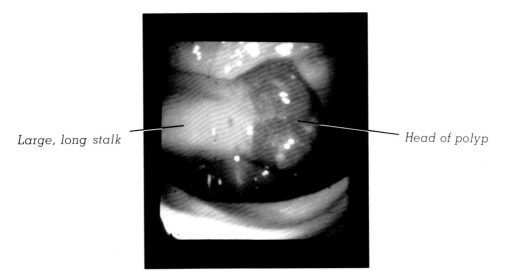

Large, long stalk   Head of polyp

Fig. 220. *Endoscopic view of a pedunculated polyp having a large, elongated stalk with a relatively small head. Disproportionate size of the head as compared to the stalk is frequently seen because of slowly developing malignancy. This change is secondary to sloughing of the polyp head. It may also be due to ischemia of the head as a result of torsion of the stalk.*

Head   Stalk   Line of resection

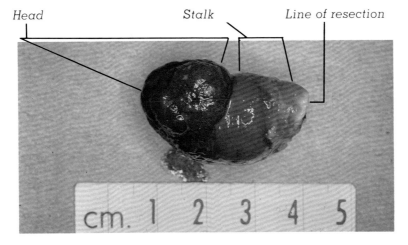

Fig. 221. *Polyp specimen (see Fig. 220) resected endoscopically shows a relatively small head and long stalk.*

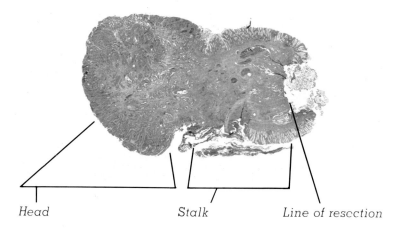

Head   Stalk   Line of resection

Fig. 222. *Histologic appearance of the same polyp (see Fig. 220).
Almost the entire head showed carcinomatous changes.*

COLONOSCOPY AND CARCINOMA OF THE COLON

Colonic carcinoma is second to lung cancer as the leading cause of death from
malignancies in the United States. In 1977, the annual new case rate was 99,000
in the United States. This disease predominates in the West, a fact that has been
attributed, in part, to a diet high in saturated fats and low in residue; nonetheless, an increasing incidence is being reported worldwide.

The possibility of a surgical cure depends on the stage of involvement. Stag-
ing is done by the Duke's classification. A Duke's A tumor refers to one limited
to the bowel wall without serosal involvement. As the classification increases
(B,C,D), so does depth of extension through the bowel wall (B), to draining
lymphatics (C) and ultimate spread to the liver and beyond (D). Cure rates of
90% or better with Duke's A lesions fall as the depth of invasion increases and
plummets with hepatic metastasis. There had been no real change in early detection of colonic carcinoma over the three decades before colonoscopy was
introduced. Although it is still too early to tell, we anticipate that colonoscopy
will alter these statistics by allowing earlier detection of carcinomas that may be
asymptomatic and by detecting and removing polyps, which we believe are
premalignant structures.

Since early detection is the key to cure in this disease, colonoscopy can, in
theory, improve survival rates. First of all, a suspicious lesion on barium enema
can be visualized directly, brushed for cytologic studies and biopsied. Furthermore, other suspicious lesions noted during the examination can also be
checked and the level noted. If a barium enema indicates a suspicious lesion on
the right or left side of the colon, colonoscopy can exclude the presence of
similar lesions on the opposite side and help guide the surgeon to the type of
operation necessary.

Because of our policy to do colonoscopy for symptomatic patients despite negative barium enemas, we have referred patients to surgery earlier with cancers that would not have been detected unless subsequent roentgenographic examination or symptoms suggested further evaluation.

Occult gastrointestinal bleeding, or anemia or both in an adult with no known source of blood loss are indications for colonoscopy. We have found many early carcinomas in this group. We, too, have found an increased rate of coexisting cancers and polyps.

Colonic carcinomas can be detected, especially in patients with rapid mucosal turnover, such as in longstanding chronic ulcerative colitis. However, some patients have synchronous tumors that were missed before resection for colorectal cancer and return several years later with a mistaken diagnosis of metachronous carcinoma. This observation emphasizes the need for colonoscopy, even if a barium enema outlines a colonic carcinoma. The exact incidence of this tumor is unknown, although the data should be forthcoming. Polyps that were not noted on x-ray films before surgical intervention for colonic carcinoma may bleed one to two years later and cause problems for the patient, even if benign. In 20%-50% of cases with colorectal carcinoma, associated polyps are found. Heald and Lockhart-Mummery noted that 60% of patients with colorectal carcinoma had a history of benign colonic tumors.

Whether benign or malignant, these small polyps or synchronous tumors are difficult to palpate during surgical procedures and are apt to be missed if colonoscopy is not done.

COLONIC POLYP
TO CARCINOMA SEQUENCE

Because of the ability to detect and remove colonic polyps, colonoscopy will probably reduce the incidence of colonic carcinoma.

Endoscopic excision of polyps with a snare-wire and electrocautery device is now widespread. Although we recognized that the procedure was potentially hazardous when we began using it in 1969, the rewards have included a better understanding of the colonic polyp-cancer sequence. The removal of a polyp in a premalignant phase is easily accomplished, although a large, bulky polyp may require segmental excision over several months. If a lesion is highly suspicious with malignant changes, immediate resection can be carried out, thus affording the patient a better chance for cure.

Recent studies have come to the fore supporting the theory that most colorectal cancers begin as polyps. Studies by Morson et al. in London, Lane et al. in New York, Enterline and Fitts et al. in Philadelphia support this contention.

The confusion that has clouded the field seems to result from an imprecise definition of polyp classifications. Lane et al. propose that 90% of all polyps are hyperplastic, not neoplastic in the true sense of the word. If we eliminate these polyps and concentrate on the neoplastic polyps, including tubular, villous and villotubular adenomas and polypoid carcinomas, we are dealing with polyps that have a malignant potential. Mason and Riddell of England and pathologists at our institution (Drs. Stenger, Mori and Chabon) are in agreement with this nomenclature and theory, and it is this classification that we use.

Adenomas clearly have the highest potential for malignant change. Using similar criteria to determine malignancy within a polyp, Grinnell and Lane, Enterline et al. and Wolff and Shinya found invasive carcinoma within a polyp approximately 5.7%-6.3% of the time. There are two problems in comparing these groups. One is that our group studied almost twice as many cases as did the other two groups, and adding all results may alter these statistics. The second is that the polyps found by our group were above the area reached by sigmoidoscopy and were removed endoscopically.

Obviously, a common definition of "malignancy" must be established before we can compare data. Although we are relying on guidelines set by Morson, Lane, Enterline and their respective coworkers, we must further establish precise definitions of carcinoma in situ and invasive carcinoma. Since carcinoma in situ does not metastasize, only invasive carcinoma should be considered malignant in the true sense of the word. Invasive carcinoma implies penetration to the muscularis mucosa. A superficial carcinoma that does not reach this level will not metastasize. The explanation of this phenomenon can be elucidated from the electron microscopy studies of Fenoglio et al. These workers demonstrated that there are no lymphatics in the colonic mucosa, only in the muscularis mucosa. Therefore, if cancer does not reach the muscularis mucosa, it cannot metastasize. Polyps without extension of carcinoma to this level are not clinically malignant. It is essential that the entire polyp be retrieved, if possible, and that adequate tissue sections be made to determine if the polyp fits the criteria for malignancy.

Several observations seem to justify the present theory of the polyp-cancer sequence:

1. Foci of severe dysplasia and frank carcinoma are frequently seen in adenomas, not in normal or hyperplastic mucosa.
2. Adenomas show abnormal cell regeneration unlike normal mucosa.
3. As polyp size increases, risk of cancer increases.
4. Polyps with severe dysplasia of the epithelium have a very high malignant potential, suggestive of a steplike progression from dysplasia to in situ carcinoma to microinvasion to invasion of the muscularis mucosa.
5. Patients with polyps have a higher incidence of carcinoma than the normal population.
6. Many carcinomas show evidence of adjacent benign or adenomatous growth, suggesting origin in the benign tissue, with rapid overgrowth as the carcinoma spreads.
7. Aggressive removal of polyps with stringent follow-up examinations can decrease the expected incidence of cancer of the rectum and rectosigmoid.

The gross pathologic appearance of colonic cancer has been described by several investigators:

Sackman (1968)
1. Scirrhous cancer
2. Colloid cancer
3. Polypoid cancer
4. Crateriform cancer

Berk (1964)

1. Nodular
2. Scirrhous
3. Mucinous or colloid
4. Papillary adenocarcinoma

Goligher (1967)

1. Polypoid or cauliflower cancer
2. Ulcerative cancer
3. Annular or stenosing cancer
4. Diffusely infiltrating cancer
5. Colloid cancer

Morson (1972)

1. Ulcerating tumors with raised everted edges
2. Protuberant type
3. Colloid appearance (cut surface)
4. Scirrhous type

Our endoscopic classification of colonic carcinoma is as follows:

1. Polypoid or fungating carcinoma
2. Discoid, ulcerating type
3. Annular, constricting, granular type
3A. Annular, constricting, fibrotic type (rare)

In a recent study of 712 patients with carcinoma of the large bowel, we performed colonoscopies over an 11-year period (1968-78). In 546 patients, the carcinoma was annular and/or ulcerating; in 148, it was polypoid. The initial colonoscopy was performed before operation in 428 patients and shortly after resection in 284.

At the initial colonoscopy, synchronous carcinomas of the colon were found in 54 (7.5%) patients and benign polyps in 316 (44.4%) patients. A total of 455 polyps were excised, of which 164 (36%) had severe dysplasia, carcinoma in situ or carcinoma superficial to the muscularis mucosa.

After surgical resection of the carcinoma, all patients were advised to return for follow-up colonoscopy at six-month intervals. Compliance with this request resulted in self-selection of this group of 712 patients into two groups. There were 341 (47.9%) patients who returned as suggested and 371 (52.1%) who neglected this advice and did not have follow-up colonoscopy.

In the group of 341 patients observed for six months to 11 years, 252 (74%) were asymptomatic, and 89 (26%) had complaints of rectal bleeding, change in bowel habits or abdominal pain. In the course of follow-up examinations, 218 (64%) of this group were found to have a total of 455 polyps. Histologic evaluation of these polyps revealed that 387 (85%) were benign, 36 (8%) had severe dysplasia and 32 (7%) had carcinoma in situ. Invasive carcinoma did not develop in any patient in this group.

In the group of 371 patients who failed to return for follow-up colonoscopy, metachronous carcinomas of the colon occurred in 33 (8.9%) patients. The incidence of carcinoma in this group of patients compared to the group with follow-up colonoscopy is statistically significant at all levels by the chi-square test (Figs. 223-231).

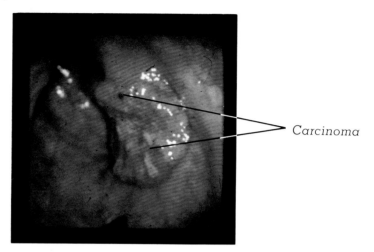

Fig. 223. Endoscopic view of an ulcerated, discoid-shaped carcinoma, measuring approximately 1.5 × 2.0, cm in the sigmoid colon.

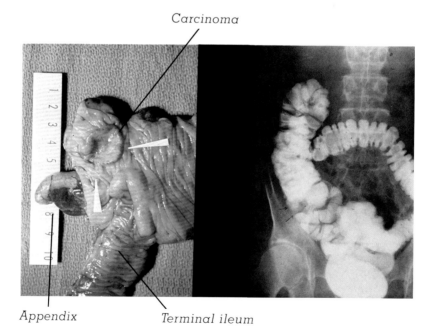

Fig. 224. A 61-year-old man with chronic anemia. A barium enema was negative (right). Endoscopy revealed an ulcerated lesion measuring 2 cm in diameter. The resected specimen is shown on the left.

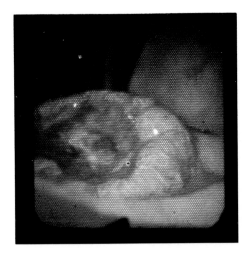

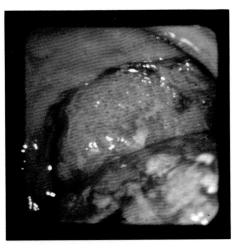

Fig. 225. Closeup endoscopic view of an ulcerated adenocarcinoma of the sigmoid measuring 1.5 cm in diameter.

Fig. 226. Endoscopic view of a large, bulky, ulcerated carcinoma in the proximal sigmoid colon.

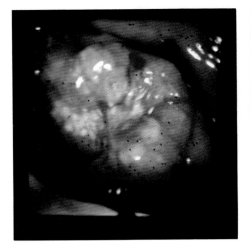

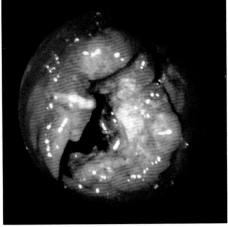

Fig. 227. Endoscopic view of a constricting, ulcerated carcinoma of the hepatic flexure.

Fig. 228. Endoscopic view of a constricting, ulcerated, annular carcinoma of the distal sigmoid colon. A barium enema was negative.

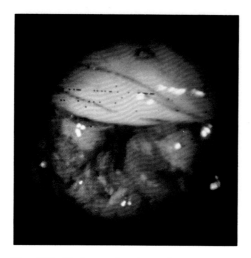 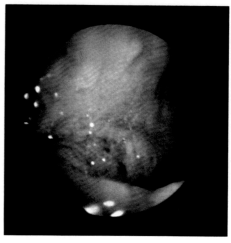

Fig. 229. *Endoscopic view of a constricting, annular carcinoma of the ileocecal junction. The lesion is partially covered by a mucosal fold.*

Fig. 230. *Endoscopic view of a carcinomatous lesion of the sigmoid. The patient had a large ovarian cancer that had invaded the colon.*

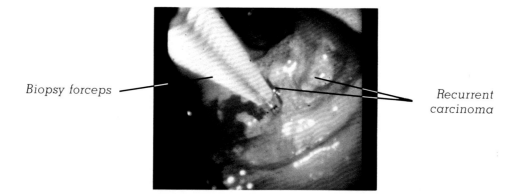

Biopsy forceps ———   Recurrent
                                                      carcinoma

Fig. 231. *Biopsy of a recurrent carcinoma at the anastomotic line of previously resected bowel.*

MULTIPLE POLYPOSIS

This term refers to the presence of numerous (but usually fewer than 100) adenomatous colonic polyps. They are frequently disseminated throughout the entire colon and are not associated with any familial syndrome. There is some suggestion that this disease may represent a variant of familial polyposis. Carcinoma of the colon in these patients is statistically higher than among healthy persons because of the great number of adenomatous polyps (Figs. 232-235).

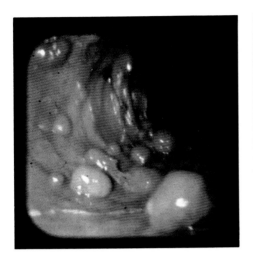

Fig. 232. *Numerous colonic polyps (adenomas) in a patient without a family history of colonic neoplasm.*

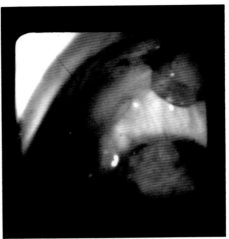

Fig. 234. *Endoscopic view of two polypoid lesions of the sigmoid. Both polyps contained partially invasive carcinoma.*

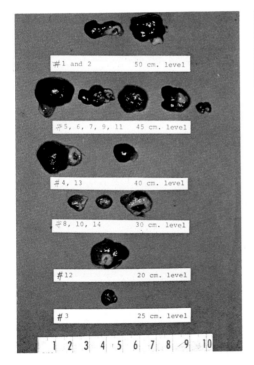

Fig. 233. *Fourteen polyps excised endoscopically from the left colon. Two polyps showed foci of invasive carcinoma. However, the patient was managed conservatively because of a history of heart disease.*

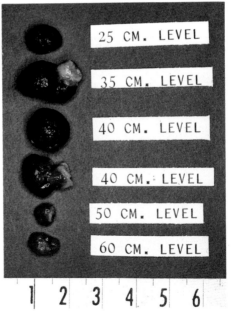

Fig. 235. *Colonic polyps excised endoscopically from the midsigmoid to the left transverse colon. The anatomic levels of the polyps should also be recorded on the chart.*

FAMILIAL POLYPOSIS

Familial polyposis is a rare generalized form of inherited polyposis. The mode of inheritance is believed to be an autosomal dominant gene with variable penetrance. The usual feature of this syndrome is the presence of numerous colonic polyps of various sizes. Hundreds of polyps, all adenomatous, are found (Figs. 236 and 237). There are no extracolonic features in this syndrome. The polyps are usually sessile; however, they may be pedunculated.

Symptoms include rectal bleeding, diarrhea, cramps and, if the diarrhea is profuse, possibly electrolyte changes.

The great danger to patients with this syndrome is malignant degeneration of the polyps. Usually, from the age of 30, the malignant potential is 100%.

The diagnosis is easily made by colonoscopy. All members of an affected patient's family should be examined.

Because of the high incidence of carcinoma of the colon, we recommend subtotal colectomy if the number or size of the polyps increases. Usually, by the age of 30, most patients should have a subtotal colectomy with ileoproctostomy or a total proctocolectomy. The rectal stump should be examined endoscopically once or twice each year, and all remaining polyps should be excised. After colectomy, many rectal polyps may regress.

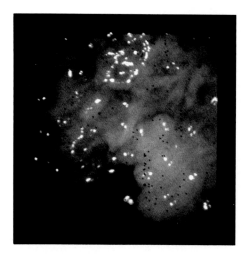 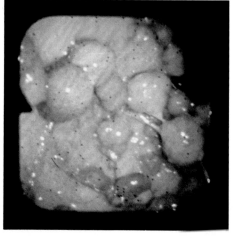

Fig. 236. Endoscopic view of familial polyposis in a 20 year-old patient. The polyps measured 0.2-0.4 cm in diameter. Subtotal colectomy was performed.

Fig. 237. Endoscopic view of familial polyposis in a 55-year-old woman. The polyps measured approximately 0.5-1.3 cm in diameter. Total proctocolectomy was performed.

An interesting variant of familial polyposis is Gardner's syndrome. Here, numerous colonic polyps are seen in association with polyps in the stomach and small bowel (Fig. 238). In addition, cutaneous and bony manifestations, such as fibromas, desmoid tumors, sebaceous cysts, osteomas and other connective tissue tumors, may be present as well. The colonic polyps, again, are adenomatous and show a 100% tendency toward malignant degeneration.

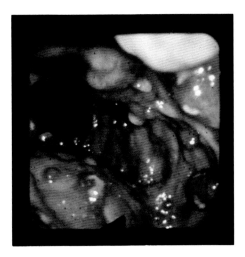

Fig. 238a. Numerous colonic polyps in a patient with Gardner's syndrome.

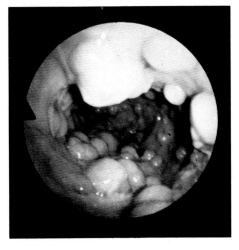

Fig. 238b. Another patient with Gardner's syndrome showing numerous colonic polyps.

12

Other Malignant Lesions

LYMPHOMA (LYMPHOSARCOMA)

Two percent of all malignant gastrointestinal tumors are lymphomas, and are rarely seen in the colon and rectum.

Colonic lymphoma may be noted at any age but is most common during the fifth to seventh decades of life. Symptoms include abdominal pain, rectal bleeding and, occasionally, signs of obstruction if the rectum is involved.

Barium enema reveals numerous findings. The lymphoma may appear as one or many mucosal or intramural growths. The lesions may involve long segments, unlike carcinoma, which is localized to short segments. Extensive involvement may appear as numerous sessile polypoid lesions widely scattered over the colon with a shaggy circumference. The diagnostic roentgenologic finding is a smooth-surfaced multinodular tumor outline. The lesion may mimic ulcerative colitis, with pseudopolyps demonstrated on barium enema.

Endoscopic Appearance

Lymphoma does not initially involve the mucosal surface, and the mucosa overlying the lesion may at first appear pale. A submucosal nodule or group of adjoining nodules may protrude into the lumen. The latter may cause the colonic surface to appear as though it had numerous large folds. Ulceration occurs when the mucosal surface becomes infiltrated. The ulcerations are different from those seen with adenocarcinoma because lymphomatous ulcers are ringed by folds or overhanging mucosal edges and resemble lopsided lunar craters (Fig. 239). Involvement of colon and mesentery can lead to intussusception. At times, the lesion may have a polypoid appearance (Fig. 240). All lesions must be biopsied for a definitive diagnosis (Fig. 241).

Lymphoma localized to the rectum has a relatively good prognosis if it is resected locally or treated with radiotherapy or if both procedures are done.

Although lymphoma is sufficiently sensitive to irradiation, external radiation may not cure the lesion because it is difficult to reach this area using such

170

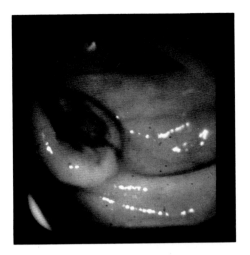

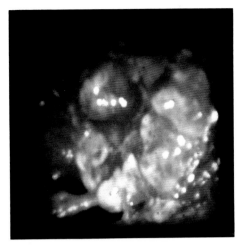

Fig. 239. Ulcerated lymphosarcoma measuring approximately 2 cm in diameter. The elevated edge of the lesions is covered with colonic mucosa and may resemble other submucosal lesions.

Fig. 240. Endoscopic view of an ulcerated, fungating, friable lymphosarcoma of the cecum. This type of lymphosarcoma is difficult to differentiate from adenocarcinoma.

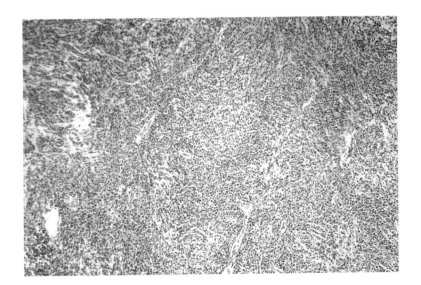

Fig. 241. Histologic appearance of a lymphosarcoma.

therapy. Endoanal techniques of delivering radiation are relatively new in this country. Therefore, several treatment modalities exist and all have places in treatment. The most important variable in determining a successful outcome is the presence of systemic disease, which, of course, necessitates systemic treatment.

MELANOMA

Malignant melanoma is a rare lesion of the lower gastrointestinal tract. It occurs most commonly in the anorectal region and appears in pigmented and nonpigmented (amelanotic) forms (Figs. 242 and 243). Malignant melanoma may also be a metastatic lesion from the skin to the gastrointestinal tract. Endoscopically, the lesions may resemble thrombosed hemorrhoids or hyperplastic polyps. They have a characteristic rubbery feeling when touched with a biopsy forceps. These lesions should not be excised endoscopically; more extensive treatment is required.

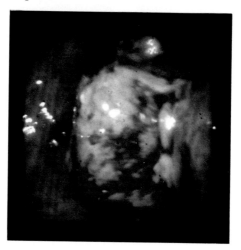

Fig. 242. Endoscopic view of a melanoma of the distal rectum measuring approximately 2 cm in diameter.

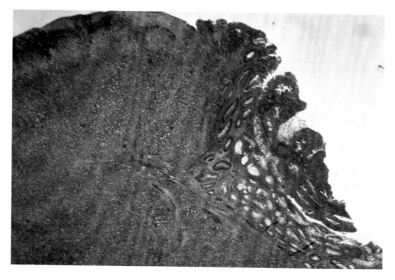

Fig. 243. Histologic appearance of a melanoma.

13

Biopsy and Cytology

Biopsy

The use of biopsy in diagnosing colonic lesions is an integral part of the endoscopy procedure. The need for tissue specimens to confirm or rule out colonic disease makes it necessary to understand how and where to biopsy.

Numerous types of biopsy forceps are available. Any standard biopsy forceps can be used. All suspicious lesions should be sampled. We prefer to use the cold biopsy forceps without coagulation. The amount of bleeding after biopsy is minimal and of little consequence.

Small lesions may be completely excised with several bites of the forceps. Large lesions should be sampled at strategic areas, such as the marginal and central zones. This approach insures that both surrounding normal mucosa and tissue in obviously diseased regions are obtained. In addition, a deep bite into the lesion should be done to obtain samples of the basement membrane and submucosa. These tissues can be obtained by repeat biopsies into the depth of a lesion. This method also allows the operator to obtain a large specimen.

Obvious carcinomas should be biopsied for tissue diagnosis. Polypoid lesions should be biopsied if they show any malignant changes. Different areas of the colon in suspected inflammatory bowel disease should be sampled to confirm the diagnosis and to rule out malignant degeneration. Areas of colonic narrowing should be biopsied as well.

Biopsy is also useful in suspected infectious diseases, such as amebiasis, where stool examination has been negative.

The forceps is passed through the biopsy channel approximately 1-2 cm past the instrument tip. The jaws are then opened and directed toward the lesion. The instrument tip usually can be advanced to the lesion without moving the forceps. However, it sometimes becomes necessary to advance the forceps.

After obtaining the specimen, the forceps is pulled back through the channel and dipped into a formalin jar, releasing the tissue. To avoid crushing or to obtain a large specimen, it is preferable to pull back the entire instrument with the forceps just outside the tip of the scope, release the specimen in a formalin jar and then retract the forceps from the biopsy channel.

Cytology

Two popular methods used for obtaining cytology specimens are brush and water lavage. Brushing is a standard method for obtaining specimens. Using a Waterpik jet to flush a suspicious area allows the operator to filter the return and examine it under the microscope.

14

Electrocautery

The use of electrocautery has become widespread in operating rooms and endoscopy suites. An understanding of the principles involved as well as a knowledge of the hazards of electrocautery are essential to the safe use of this instrument.

Ohm's law ($I = E/R$, where I is current in amps, E is voltage and R is resistance of tissue in ohms) is the major dictum controlling heat resistance of tissues. One of two types of generators is used, either a spark gap or a radiofrequency oscillator. Active and indifferent electrodes are used. The indifferent electrode, or grounding plate, must be large enough to have good skin contact, since current is discharged from the body through this pathway. The active electrode is usually small, with heat being concentrated at its tip.

Electrocautery produces either a cutting or coagulating result. Cutting occurs when high-frequency wave forms cause vaporization of tissues. Coagulation of tissue is a process of denaturation caused by damping current flow.

Coagulation of tissue is also a function of the diameter of the snare-wire, the thickness of the tissue and the traction placed on the snare-wire by an assistant.

The greater the diameter of the snare-wire, the slower it will cut through the tissue, and vice versa. The thicker the tissue, the greater the resistance and the more the current that is necessary for coagulation. Strong traction on the ensnared tissue allows for rapid transection, whereas weak traction allows for increased resistance of the coagulated tissues and thus increases cutting time. A 5-mm stalk requires approximately 3-5 seconds for transection. A short, thick stalk more than 5 mm in diameter requires adjustment of transection time while observing the extent of the burn to the base of the polyp and colonic wall. This adjustment can be made using intermittent bursts on the foot pedal of the cautery while an assistant continually places traction on the snare-wire.

The cutting current is never used. However, some endoscopists prefer a combination of cutting and coagulating current (blend). The electrocautery equipment, including connections, grounding plate and circuit, should be checked each day. The amount of current used can be checked by sparking the active electrode to the grounding plate. This check should be done on a daily basis to insure that settings are properly adjusted and that all circuits are intact. Surface contact of the ground plate to the patient must be insured. During polypectomy, only the coagulation current (set on "pure") is used.

Complications

Shock

The snare-wire is usually insulated with a polyethylene sheath. In addition, the operator wears rubber gloves. Any exposed wire is folded into the gloved hand during coagulation to prevent shock or burn. Metallic parts of the cautery instrument should not be touched during application of current.

Prevention of shock or burn to the patient is assured by proper placement of the grounding plate under a broad body surface area (e.g., exposed thigh).

Perforation (see page 203)

Perforation by electric current can occur, as noted above, when a small surface area of the polyp is in contact with the colonic wall. This allows for high concentration of electric current at one point and leads to perforation. As noted, perforation can be prevented by oscillating the polyp head. There is no danger of perforation with large polyps in contact with several areas of the colonic wall because the current is not concentrated at one point.

Hemorrhage (see page 206)

This complication occurs more often if the coagulation current is not used.

At times, a large or arteriosclerotic vessel may not coagulate well and is the cause of pulsatile bleeding. In such cases, the exposed stalk should be immediately resnared and strangulated for approximately 15-30 minutes, then slowly released. Recoagulation should not be attempted; rather, the adjacent tissues should be allowed to become edematous. This approach allows compression of bleeding vessels.

Explosion

There is no danger of gas explosion in a properly prepared bowel. Carbon dioxide insufflation to dilute combustible gases, such as hydrogen and methane, is no longer practiced.

By avoiding the use of electrocautery in a poorly prepared bowel, the risk of an explosion will be eliminated.

15

Colonoscopic Polypectomy

When a colonic polyp is detected by barium enema or colonoscopy, polypectomy should be done to assure that an invasive malignant tumor is not present. Because there is strong evidence of a premalignant potential for colonic polyps, removing benign neoplastic polyps is prophylaxis against malignant degeneration. The procedure of choice for removing colorectal polyps has been the technique of snare-cautery resection via the colonoscope, introduced in 1969. This procedure has proven reliable and accurate and is now accepted worldwide. It should be emphasized that endoscopic removal of colonic polyps should be attempted only after the operator has acquired considerable training in and experience with the technique of diagnostic colonoscopy. Colonoscopic polypectomy can replace the conventional transabdominal approach to most colonic polyps, but it must be done on the basis of sound judgment.

Colonoscopic polypectomy can be performed in an outpatient or inpatient setting. The decision between these two alternatives depends on the size and nature of the polyps, the patient's general condition and the operator's preference.

Hospitalization is recommended for patients with hypertension, diseases of the heart, liver, kidney or lung, arteriosclerosis or diabetes and for those undergoing anticoagulant therapy, including long-term aspirin intake. It is also recommended for obese patients; personal preference determines whether it is recommended for patients older than 65 years or younger than seven years.

PREPARATION OF A HOSPITALIZED PATIENT

1. Medical history
2. Physical examination
3. Complete blood count and blood chemistry
4. Urinalysis
5. Chest x-ray film and electrocardiogram
6. Screening for coagulation defects
7. Blood cross-matching and typing, if necessary

8. Informed written consent
9. Psychologic preparation

The importance of explaining the procedure to the patient cannot be overemphasized, since an understanding allays apprehensions and provides comfort for patients.

GENERAL CONSIDERATIONS

The procedure is done with the patient in the left lateral recumbent position. The operator should have at least one experienced assistant available and a teaching or lecture endoscope available. If a complete diagnostic colonoscopy has not been previously done, it is carried out, when feasible, before proceeding with polypectomy, since many patients suspected of having one polyp actually have many polyps on complete examination. When the endoscope has been advanced to the polyp, the operator should proceed if the bowel is well prepared. If there is fecal matter or fluid in the field, excision should be postponed and the bowel preparation repeated. The colonoscope is advanced approximately 25 cm beyond the level of the polyp to insure that the bowel is clean and that fecal fluid will not spill on the operative field during polypectomy. If, for any reason, the polyp cannot be well visualized, the patient's position should be altered. Once the polyp is clearly visible, the operator should quickly determine its size, shape and nature and determine the best way to remove it. The polyp can be gently manipulated with the tip of the endoscope or the snare-cautery device, if necessary, to determine whether it is sessile or pedunculated. The size, width and length of the stalk are factors that also help determine the operative approach that is undertaken.

SNARE-CAUTERY DEVICE

There are two types of snare-cautery devices. One is made of teflon tubing and a strand of braided wire folded back on itself (Fig. 244). The second, a commercial snare, is manufactured by Olympus, ACMI and Fujinon (Figs. 245 and 246). The former, a homemade snare, is safer because the tension applied to the wire can be felt more sensitively by the trained assistant than it can through the hand grip of a commercial snare. If the wire becomes stuck in the base of the stalk of the polyp during transection of the polyp, the operator may wish to discontinue cauterization without completing transection of the tissue or the stalk. With the homemade snare, the wire can be removed easily. By contrast, with the commercial snare, the wire cannot be removed, and laparotomy may be required. With the homemade snare, the size and shape of the loop can be precisely adjusted for each polyp to be excised.

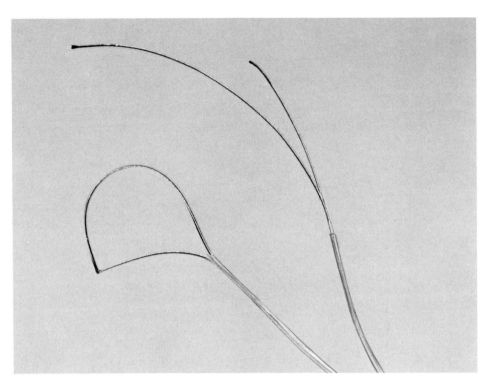

Fig. 244. *Homemade snare-wire shows loop and tail portions.*

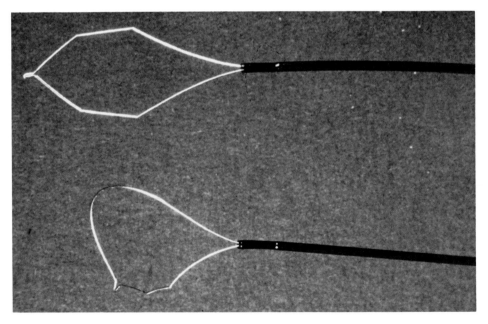

Fig. 245. *Commercial type snare-wire illustrates the various shapes of the snare-wire loop.*

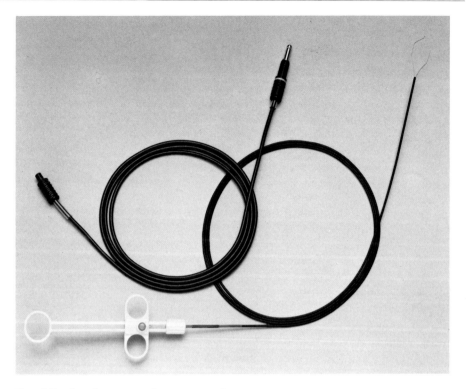

Fig. 246. Another type of commercial snare-wire.

ELECTROSURGICAL UNITS

The operator must be completely familiar with the cauterization characteristics of the device being used. It should be tested on a laboratory animal or, less reliably, on some raw meat. Electrosurgical units are made by ACMI, Bovie, Cameron Miller, Elmed, Olympus and Valley Laboratories.

POLYPECTOMY TECHNIQUE

Small Polyps Less than 0.5 cm in Diameter

Such polyps may be completely excised with several bites of the biopsy forceps, and the base coagulated after biopsy specimens are taken. An alternative method is to use the hot biopsy forceps to remove the polyps completely with coagulation.

Small Sessile Polyps Less than 1.0 cm in Diameter

Small sessile polyps can be removed by the standard snare-cautery technique if the base is not wide. The polyp is lassoed with the snare-wire, then the Teflon catheter tip is advanced to the base of the polyp to the exact point where the transection is desired (Fig. 247). The wire is then gently tightened. The polyp is gently tented toward the lumen, and the coagulation current is applied (Fig. 248).

If the base is transected too rapidly, before coagulation is adequate, bleeding may occur. However, bleeding is usually negligible, and perforation from excessive coagulation is a much more serious complication.

In applying the snare-wire to small lesions, it is important not to include normal colonic mucosa in the snare loop. When normal tissue is included, there is much more resistance to transecting the tissue than when coagulating through the polyp (Fig. 249). Increased resistance should be a warning to immediately release the snare loop and carefully examine the site of coagulation. This situation can be avoided by using the principal technique described previously.

If the polyp is snared correctly, it is easily removed by tenting the mucosa. However, if the mucosa around the polyp is caught, it is difficult to oscillate the polyp to and fro, and the wall of the colon moves.

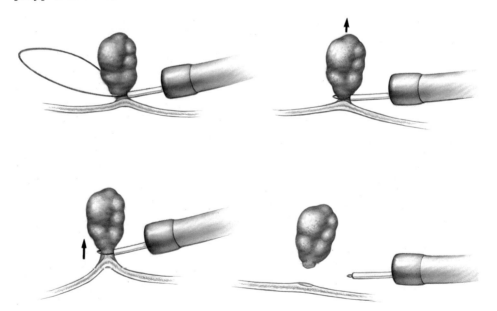

Fig. 247.

a: A wire loop is made, and the catheter tip is advanced to the neck of the polyp.

b: The loop is tightened loosely while the polyp is tented slightly to the center of the lumen. If extra mucosa is caught in the loop, it may be released at this time.

c: The wire loop is fully tightened, and the polyp is tented to the center of the lumen during cautery transection.

d: The polyp is transected in 2-3 seconds (as soon as mucosal blanching is noted) to prevent extension of the cautery burn through the bowel wall.

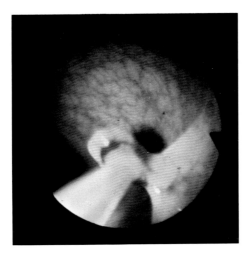

Fig. 248. *Endoscopic view of a small sessile polyp with a snare-wire encircling the base of the polyp. After the polyp is snared, it is pulled toward the center of the lumen before transection.*

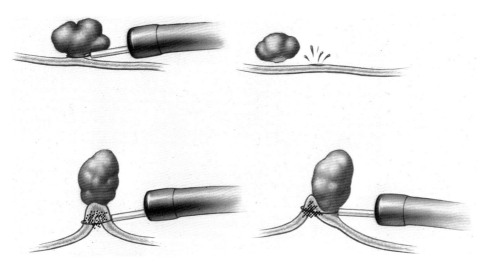

Fig. 249. *Complications of excision.*
a: A wire loop is placed around the base of the polyp, tightened and excised with cautery. If transection occurs before coagulation is adequate, minimal bleeding may result. However, in general, too little cauterization is better than too much.

b: The bowel wall is partially caught with the wire loop. The normal mucosa adjacent to the polyp is ensnared. Increased resistance to transection warns the operator that normal tissue is being cauterized. These conditions may result in transmural burns and perforation.

If the base is broad or if the polyp is larger than 1.0 cm, it must be removed piecemeal; in such cases, more than one session may be needed. It is best to remove too little rather than too much in difficult cases. The operator can return at a later session to remove additional tissue, if necessary.

Pedunculated Polyps

Polyps with Long Stalks

When removing a pedunculated polyp with a long stalk, the operator should leave at least 1.0 cm of stalk to insure safety after coagulation and to avoid perforation. Also, if bleeding occurs after transection of the stalk, this portion of the stalk can easily be resnared to achieve hemostasis. Care should be taken not to tighten the snare-wire until it has been positioned precisely at the proposed plane of resection. Care must also be taken to avoid prolonged application of current during transection to prevent burning the bowel wall (Fig. 250).

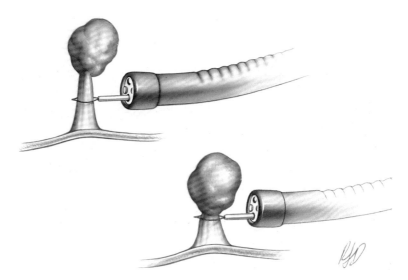

Fig. 250. Excision of a pedunculated polyp.
a: A wire loop is placed toward the neck of the polyp. Even a long remnant of stalk may be left behind without fear of recurrence. If pulsatile bleeding occurs, a long stalk is easy to resnare.
b: If there is a relatively short stalk, the snare should be brought up to the neck of the polyp.

Polyps with Short Stalks

For removing a pedunculated polyp with a short stalk, the snare should be placed as close as possible to the neck of the polyp. The snare can be placed very close by not completely tightening the wire after lassoing the polyp but, rather, leaving it slightly loose and by then positioning the tip of the teflon catheter near the neck of the polyp, before finally tightening and strangulating (Figs. 251-254).

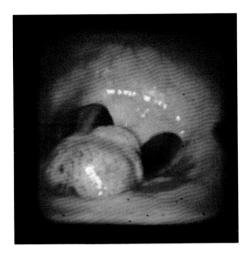

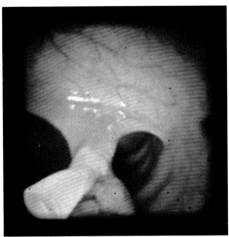

Fig. 251. *Endoscopic view of a pedunculated polyp on a short stalk. The head of the polyp measures approximately 1.5 cm in diameter.*

Fig. 252. *Endoscopic view of polypectomy. The snare-wire is placed around the neck of the polyp (same polyp as in Fig. 251.*

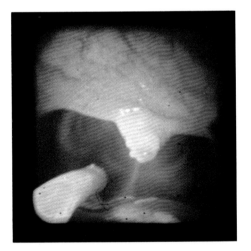

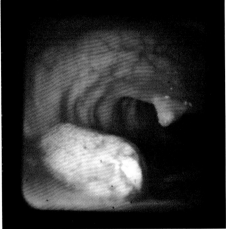

Fig. 253. *Photograph taken immediately after transection of the stalk. Observe the site of polypectomy for several seconds to confirm adequate hemostasis.*

Fig. 254. *After a period of observation, insufflated air in the proximal loop of the colon is aspirated, and the specimen is withdrawn.*

Some authorites recommend strangulating the stalk of a pedunculated polyp before applying electric current. This approach is both unnecessary and dangerous. It can result in premature transection before electric current can be applied, leading to hemorrhage and loss of visualization. In fact, the operator may lose sight of the polyp during the strangulation. It is not necessary to

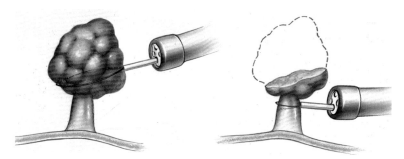

Fig. 255. Excision of a large pedunculated polyp.

a: If a polyp is a large and lobulated polyp, the wire loop may become caught in its head. Once the wire loop is tightened, the polyp should be partially excised. Otherwise, by releasing a tightened snare, the cut tissue may hemorrhage substantially, possibly obscuring the operative field.

b: After partial resection of the head, the wire loop is placed safely around the neck, and the polyp is excised completely.

strangulate the polyp for more than a few seconds before applying coagulation current. Prolonged strangulation of the polyp can also induce local spasms of the colon, and visualization of the polypectomy field may be lost.

Once the snare has been tightened on the polyp head, it should not be released or repositioned on the stalk. If it is loosened, the tissue that has been cut through with the wire will bleed and obscure the field of operation. Therefore, once the snare-wire has been applied and tightened on the polyp head, that portion of the polyp should be transected using coagulation current. After partial polypectomy, the snare is repositioned in the proper place on the stalk, and the polypectomy is completed (Fig. 255).

Polyps with Large Heads

For removing pedunculated polyps with large heads, it is necessary to reduce the size of the polyp head by segmental resection to visualize the stalk for complete polypectomy. Such polyps are usually villous or papillary (Fig. 256).

During segmental resection of a large head of a pedunculated polyp, it is necessary to avoid pulling the polyp because the stalk will be thinned out, and both the stalk and the head of the polyp may become coagulated. The operator may be unaware of this complication, and perforation may occur. Perforation can be prevented by slightly and continouously oscillating the polyp head during the segmental resection in piecemeal fashion.

Broad-Based, Pedunculated Polyps

In removing a broad-based, pedunculated polyp, the major risk is that the plane of transection will be too close to the bowel wall. If this is the case, coagulation may be transmitted to the entire colonic wall before the thick-stalked polyp is transected. It is better to remove such a polyp piecemeal or during several segmental resections (Fig. 257). These maneuvers require skill and experience.

If the entire stalk is well visualized and it is judged that the polyp can be

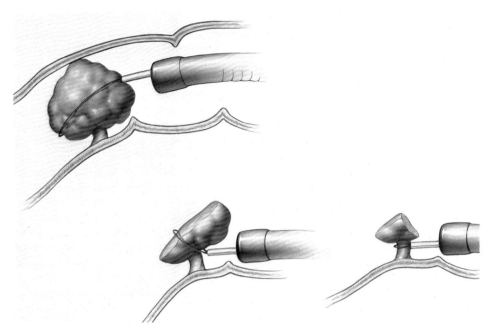

Fig. 256. Segmental excision of a large pedunculated polyp with a short stalk.

a: If the polyp is large, obscuring the stalk, the head should be excised segmentally. This approach allows satisfactory visualization of the stalk. A large portion of the polyp head is being excised. Care is taken not to pull the head of the polyp because it might thin out, coagulating the entire stalk. This response may lead to perforation during resection of the large segment of polyp.

b: Further excision of the head.

c: The stalk is now easily visualized and ensnared at the neck.

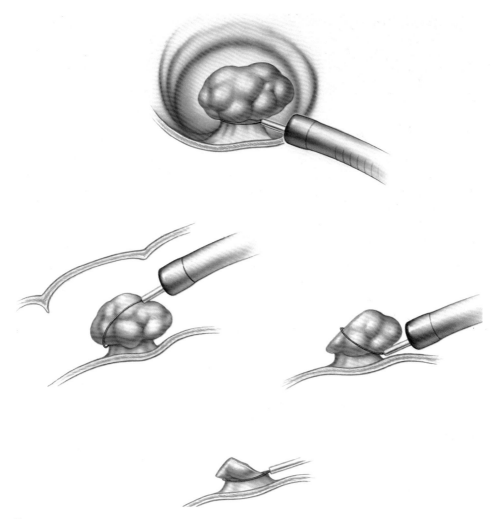

Fig. 257. *Excision of a polyp on a short, wide stalk.*
a: *If an adequate length of stalk is visualized, the wire loop may be placed around the neck of the polyp.*
b and **c:** *In cases where the stalk is not* *well visualized, or adequate length is not obtained, segmental excision of the head must be performed.*
d: *Complete excision carried out to the neck of the polyp, in a segmental fashion.*

excised safely in one segment, the snare should be passed completely around and tightened at the neck of the polyp and transection done. If, however, the operator cannot visualize the stalk completely, the polyp should be removed in a piecemeal fashion, as described previously.

Large Sessile Polyps

In patients with sessile polyps having a diameter greater than 2.0 cm, the age, general condition of the patient and the pathologic nature of the polyp help determine whether it should be managed solely by endoscopic resection or whether transabdominal resection is indicated. If the colonoscopic examination reveals that the lesion is not a grossly invasive tumor, the next step is to remove a large portion of the polyp to determine its pathologic nature. Large villous adenomas can remain completely benign for many years. To obtain as much tissue as possible safely, the polyp should be excised in a segmental fashion, as illustrated (Fig. 258).

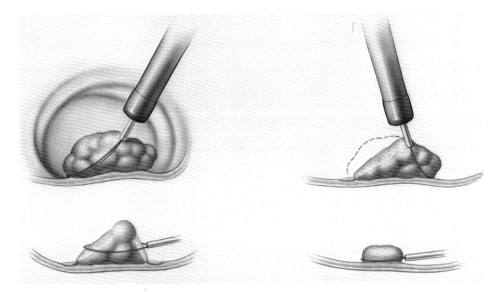

Fig. 258. Segmental excision of a large, wide-based, sessile polyp.
a: Partial excision of the head by oblique ensnarement of a large segment. A small mucosal ulceration is produced at the end of the cut.
b: The second cut is made opposite to the first cut, again leaving a small mucosal ulceration. Further excisions are performed to reduce the size of the head in a similar fashion.

c: Any remaining polypoid tissue is en- snared without transecting the base of the polyp. Too little resection during the first session is better than too much resection. Further need for resection depends on the histologic nature of the polyp.
d: After 6-8 weeks, the mucosal ulcera- tions heal, narrowing the base of the polyp. This area may be transected safely at this time. Complete excision may require more than two or three ses- sions, depending on the size of the polyp.

Because of the danger of a transmural burn, if the operator completely ensnares and coagulates a large, wide-based, sessile polyp larger than 2.0 cm in diameter, the polyp must be excised in a segmental or piecemeal fashion. The procedure is as follows (Fig. 259): the polyp is first well visualized, then a wire loop is made that encircles the base of the polyp at one end. The snare is tightened down over the polyp in an oblique plane. This approach insures that only a portion of the polyp will be transected with a small part of its base. A small mucosal ulceration will then result at the site of transection of the base (Fig. 260). This process is repeated by lying the wire loop over the opposite end

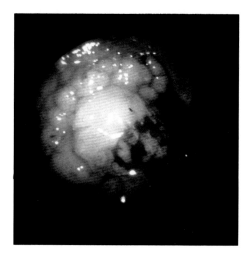

Fig. 259. *Endoscopic view of a large, lobulated, sessile polyp (villous type).*

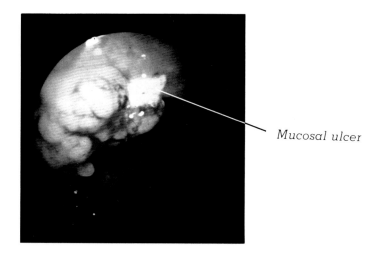

Mucosal ulcer

Fig. 260. *Same polyp shown in Fig. 259. One side is excised, resulting in traumatic ulceration of the mucosa.*

of the polyp, again in an oblique plane and at a right angle to the first cut (Fig. 261). Again, a portion of the polyp and a small part of its base will be transected, leaving a mucosal ulceration at the base. The central portion of the polyp can then be ensnared completely above the base and transected, leaving a small

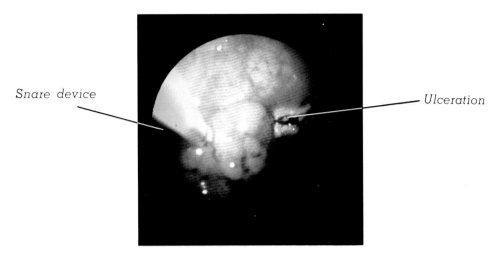

Snare device

Ulceration

Fig. 261. *Excision of additional segments of the polyp shown in Fig. 260.*

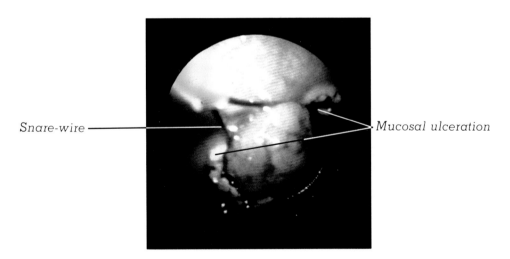

Snare-wire

Mucosal ulceration

Fig. 262. *Further excision of the polyp shown in Fig. 261.*

remnant (Fig. 262). As emphasized, it is better to take too little than too much tissue at this session. In this fashion, the base of the polyp will be narrowed, and 70%-90% of the polyp can be excised (Fig. 263).

If the polyp is benign, the remainder of the base can be removed in later

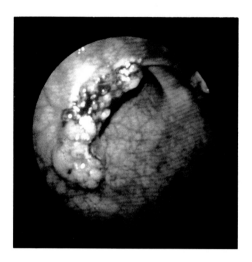

Fig. 263. Same polyp shown in Fig. 262. Approximately 80% of the lesion has now been excised. If the histologic features show that the polyp is benign, it can be excised completely in about 3-6 weeks.

sessions. Similar oblique cuts are made through the base of the polyp, which has scarred, leaving a narrow-based, sessile polyp. The polyp can now be completely ensnared and transected at its base. As mentioned, these procedures should be carried out at several sessions at three- to four-week intervals. I cannot emphasize enough the importance of excising too little tissue rather than too much. This approach avoids perforation of the colonic wall.

Removal of sessile polyps is more complicated than is removal of pedunculated polyps in that the margin of transection and cauterization is always directly on the bowel wall. The endoscopic appearance of a sessile polypoid lesion is the single most important variable in deciding whether a lesion can be removed colonoscopically. In general, colonoscopic polypectomy should be considered only for benign sessile lesions that are soft, smooth, velvety and lobulated. Lesions larger than 3.0 cm in diameter are sometimes removed endoscopically, but in such cases the operator must be experienced in endoscopic morphology and electrosurgery techniques.

Malignant sessile polypoid lesions are generally firm, granular and friable and may also be ulcerated. A large sessile polypoid lesion should always be managed by colectomy, provided, of course, that the patient's general condition permits. Although size, location and radiographic appearance of a polypoid lesion are important considerations, they do not compare with the accuracy of the information provided by direct visualization of the lesion by colonoscopy.

Polypectomy in Patients with Pacemakers

We have had considerable experience with polypectomy in patients with both temporary and permanent pacemakers. By monitoring both pulse and electrocardiographic complexes during polypectomy, we have noted no change in pulse rate or quality, although electrical interference is seen on the oscilloscope during coagulation. This pattern returns to normal when coagulation is terminated. It must be remembered, however, that the time required for coagulation ranges from several seconds to a maximum of 10 seconds.

There should be no difficulty doing electrocoagulation through a colonoscope for polypectomy or fulguration in a patient with a pacemaker as long as the settings are in standard range and the procedure is carried out in an expedient manner.

Retrieving the Specimen

The tip of the instrument is placed flush against the head of the polyp, and suction is applied. The polyp is retrieved by withdrawing the colonoscope. The operator must be careful not to apply suction too early before the head of the polyp is against the tip of the colonoscope. Otherwise, the mucosa will be suctioned. In addition, if the specimen is lost, it can be retrieved by passing the polypectomy site with the tip of the colonoscope and then injecting 1,000-2,000 ml of water or saline through the instrument. The colonoscope is then withdrawn as air is aspirated from the colon. The patient then usually passes the specimen along with the water into the bed pan (Fig. 264).

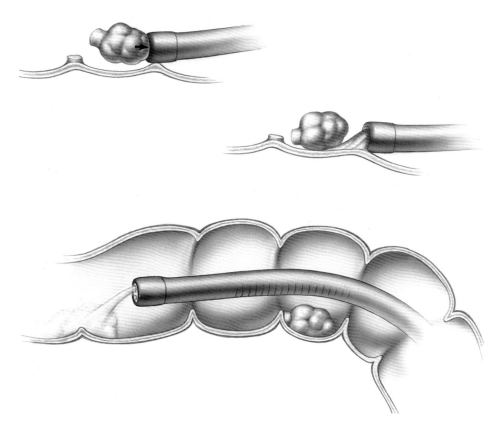

Fig. 264. *Retrieval of a polyp after excision.*
a: Suction is applied to the polyp specimen when the instrument tip comes in complete contact with its surface.
b: Inadvertent suctioning before contact with the specimen may result in mucosal aspiration and reddening out, prevent- *ing retrieval of the polyp.*
c: For retrieval of lost polyp specimens, 1-2 liters of water or saline is injected proximal to the area of polypectomy, and the colonoscope is withdrawn while air is aspirated. Enema fluid is then evacuated, along with the specimen, into a bedpan and retrieved.

When retrieving large specimens, it is sometimes difficult to use the suction method. The polyp may be squeezed by the colonic lumen and also may have trouble getting through the anal canal. For this reason, we usually lasso such polyps with a wire loop and try to snare them around the stalk area. This area is usually firmer, and there is less risk of cutting through the polyp specimen. The polyp is then withdrawn. When the anal canal is reached, the specimen is brought up flush to the tip of the instrument as the patient strains. This approach usually forces out the instrument along with the polyp (Fig. 265).

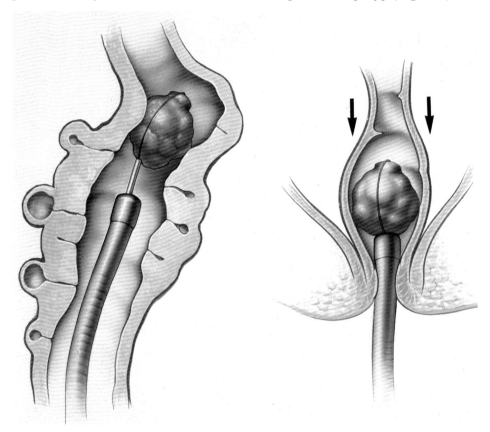

Fig. 265. *Retrieval of a specimen of a polyp measuring more than 2.5 cm in diameter.*
a: A large specimen may be squeezed off the colonic lumen, especially in a narrowed segment of the sigmoid. The snare-wire can be applied around the specimen. Approximately 2 cm are main- *tained between the snared specimen and the tip of the colonoscope to allow visualization of the lumen.*
b: When the ensnared specimen is brought to the anus, it is pulled to the tip of the colonoscope, then the patient is asked to bear down, thereby evacuating the instrument along with the specimen.

Removing Multiple Polyps Endoscopically

Multiple colonic polyps can be removed either in one or several sessions. However, if a patient has polyps scattered throughout the colon on the left and right sides, it is preferable to divide the excisions into two sessions (Fig. 266). In this way, if there is any postoperative complication, such as bleeding or perforation, the area where the complication has occurred can be easily localized. Patients with as many as 50 colonic polyps that prove benign can have them all resected through the colonoscope avoiding operative resection.

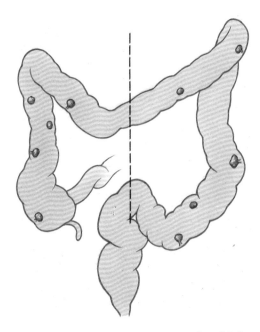

Fig. 266. *Endoscopic excision of multiple polyps. When several polyps are present throughout the entire colon, they should be evaluated for any gross malignant changes. If they are all benign in appearance, the colon is divided into left and right segments. These areas are treated during separate sessions 3-6 weeks apart. In this way, any complications that arise are easily located, and appropriate surgical management is carried out.*

Retrieving Multiple Specimens Using a Splinting Device

Retrieving multiple specimens or polyps in the right, or transverse colon is time-consuming and, occasionally, difficult. In such cases, the long colonoscope is first inserted with the splinting device; after the splint is put in place, the long colonoscope is withdrawn, and the short instrument may be inserted. The latter is then passed easily to the transverse, or right colon, where the polyps are excised. The polyps can be easily retrieved, and the colonoscope reinserted with the splinting device in place, so that a redundant sigmoid does not have to be traversed many times (Fig. 267).

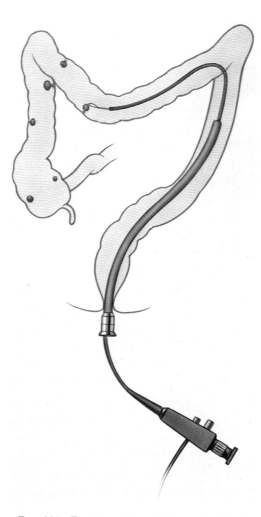

Fig. 267. *Excision of multiple right-sided colonic polyps using the splinting device. To excise several right-sided polyps and retrieve the specimens, the splinting device is left in place. The colonoscope may then be easily and repeatedly inserted through a difficult sigmoid colon.*

16

Endoscopic Management of Polyps (Adenomas) Showing Malignant Degeneration

Management of Polyps with Dysplasia or Carcinoma in Situ (mucosal carcinoma)

Most clinicians and pathologists agree that whatever the premalignant potential of precancerous or cancerous change in the mucosa of an adenoma, excision of the entire lesion eliminates the need for further concern, particularly if there has been no penetration of the muscularis mucosa. We concur with this doctrine.

If a pedunculated or a narrow-based sessile polyp has been completely excised endoscopically and shows some evidence of dysplasia or carcinoma in situ, no further resection is required. On the other hand, if a wide-based sessile polyp cannot be excised completely and there is evidence of dysplasia or carcinoma in situ, we usually recommend that a segmental bowel resection be performed in younger patients. For elderly patients or those in poor medical condition, we elect to treat them conservatively and do colonoscopy at frequent intervals (approximately 3-6 months) to determine if invasive carcinoma is present. Frequent endoscopic resections and fulgurations may lead to complete excision of such lesions. The key determinants are:

1. Nature and extent of the local pathologic changes
2. Age and general medical condition of the patient

Management of Adenomas with Invasive Carcinoma and Polypoid Tumor (malignant polyps)

Colonoscopic polypectomy is still a relatively new technique. We are currently collecting data to help determine definitive management for malignant polyps. Our initial approach was based on data accumulated from the removal of

195

polyps through the sigmoidoscope, since higher lesions were removed by colotomy or segmental colectomy.

Most authorities believe that even when a malignant tumor penetrates through the muscularis mucosa, endoscopic polypectomy is sufficient if there is an adequate zone of clearance between the plane of resection and the level of invasion. This is particularly true of pedunculated lesions. In general, we also agree with this concept. Although some case reports have described colonic wall involvement or distant lymphatic metastases (or both), such cases are rare.

In our polypectomy series, 345 patients had adenomas with invasive carcinoma, and 73 had polypoid carcinomas. Of these malignant polyps, 172 were observed more than three years. Ninety-seven were treated by colonoscopic polypectomy only because of various clinical reasons, including age of the patient, high surgical risk and associated malignant disease. There were two local recurrences of polypoid carcinomas in the initial six to 12 weeks of follow-up examinations. These small (2-3 mm) recurrent lesions were again excised endoscopically, and follow-up studies did not demonstrate any further recurrence. No other patients showed evidence of local or distal recurrence. Among the 172 patients with malignant polyps, 75 underwent colonic resection after endoscopic polypectomy. In three patients, small residual tumors were found in the surgical specimens. In two of these three patients, residual tumor was suspected preoperatively on endoscopic examination; the other patient had a microscopic focus of residual tumor (Fig. 268). In only one patient in this surgical series was an adjacent metastatic lymph node found in the pericolic region.

Our experience also militates against recommending abdominal surgery for

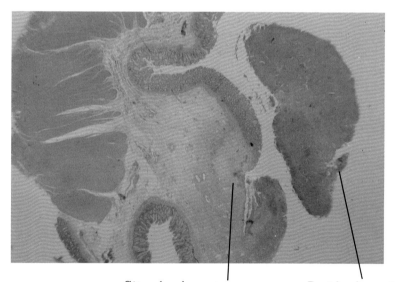

Site of polypectomy   Residual carcinoma

Fig. 268. *Histologic appearance of a specimen resected surgically 2 weeks after endoscopic polypectomy. A small residual carcinoma is seen.*

all patients with malignant polyps. When a malignant lesion extends to or is close to the cauterized tissue, the operator must consider the possibility that all malignant tissue has not been excised. Our policy under such circumstances is to recommend colectomy for good-risk patients (Figs. 269-271).

In patients with polypoid carcinoma, we are not convinced that endoscopic excision completely fulfills the accepted criteria for adequate cancer surgery and therefore advise surgical intervention for such patients. However, exceptions should be made when there is a long stalk, for the elderly or other poor-risk patients and for patients who refuse an operation. The risks of surgical intervention in elderly patients and those with complicating diseases are carefully weighed against the risk of the possibility of residual carcinoma and lymphatic metastasis.

In summary, the absolute indications for colonic resection after excision of malignant polyps are:

1. Any residual malignant tumor that is recognized endoscopically
2. Malignant changes that involve the line of resection
3. Any evidence of lymphatic or vascular involvement in the excised specimen
4. Carcinoma that is poorly differentiated cytologically (rare)

A relative indication is malignant degeneration close to the line of resection.

When no surgical intervention is recommended, colonoscopy offers considerable advantage in permitting the polypectomy site to be reexamined every few months.

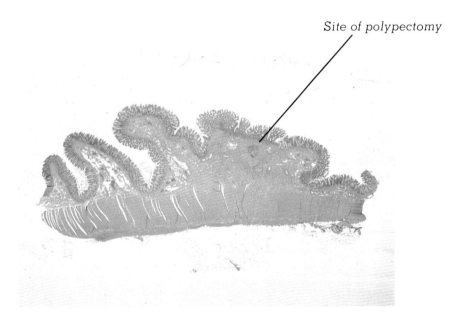

Site of polypectomy

Fig. 269. Histologic appearance of another specimen resected surgically. No residual carcinoma is seen.

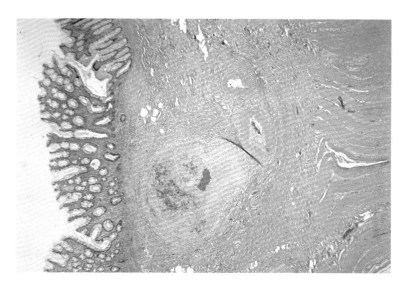

Fig. 270. High-power view of a histologic section of the specimen shown in Fig. 269.

Residual stalk

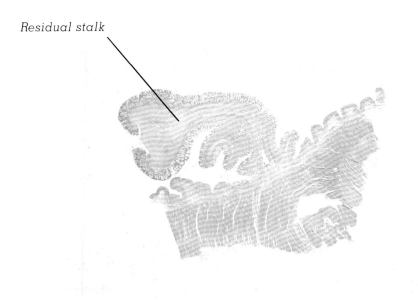

Fig. 271. Segment of colon resected surgically after endoscopic excision of a pedunculated polyp that contained invasive carcinoma.

17

Complications:
Prevention
and Management

The advantages of colonoscopy and colonoscopic polypectomy have received much publicity during the past several years. Little attention, however, has been given to associated complications or their prevention and management.

In 1975 and 1978, two surveys were conducted to determine the incidence of complications from colonoscopy and polypectomy. Statistics were collected for the American Society of Colon and Rectal Surgeons (ASCRS) and the American Society of Gastrointestinal Endoscopy (ASGE) (Table 12).

Table 12. Complications of Colonoscopy

	ASGE	*ASCRS*
Perforation		
Diagnostic	25,298(0.22%)	12,746(0.3%)
Polypectomy	6,214(1.9%)	7,393(0.5%)
Hemorrhage		
Diagnostic (%)	0.05	0.07
Polypectomy (%)	1.8	1.0
Deaths (%)	0.03	

The two major complications from colonoscopy and polypectomy are perforation and hemorrhage. The incidence of these complications is less than 1%, particularly in large series reported by experienced colonoscopists. However, the rate is close to 1% in series described by newly trained or inexperienced colonoscopists.

DIAGNOSTIC COLONOSCOPY

Cardiopulmonary Complications

In a cardiac patient, the bowel should be prepared with care to avoid dehydration, hypovolemia or water intoxication. These conditions may lead to myocardial infarction and cardiac failure.

Respiratory depression or arrest is almost always caused by overdose and/or rapid administration of an intravenous sedative, such as meperidine or diazepam. Elderly patients, especially those over 70 years of age, are particularly susceptible. For these patients, meperidine (50 mg), with or without diazepam (5 mg), are the drugs of choice; these doses should not be exceeded.

The intravenous injection should be given slowly over 30 seconds. An overdose of meperidine or diazepam also produces cardiopulmonary depression. If a patient is cyanotic or unresponsive, naloxone (0.4-0.8 mg) should be given immediately by the intravenous route to reverse the meperidinel effect; respiratory assistance with oxygen should be given as well.

Phlebitis

Thrombophlebitis is a well-recognized complication that occurs when diazepam is injected rapidly into a small vein. Selection of a large vein for injection, and flushing of the vein with 5-10 ml of normal saline immediately after injection of diazepam, may prevent this complication.

Perforation

Perforation during diagnostic colonoscopy is most often caused by overly vigorous insertion of the instrument. An inexperienced colonoscopist should use a smaller dose of medication, and the level of discomfort should be monitored carefully. When advancement of the colonoscope meets with resistance, or the patient has considerable discomfort, the endoscopist should discontinue further insertion of the instrument.

In such cases, fluoroscopy may be helpful. Marked "bowing" of a colonoscope in a loop of colon, or "looping" of the bowel, can be identified, released and straightened by turning the instrument under fluoroscopy. Advancement of a colonoscope against resistance should never be attempted, even if the colonic lumen can be seen.

Vigorous rotational motion may also result in perforation by tearing the bowel wall. The key to successful and safe introduction of the instrument is the ability to visualize the colonic lumen at all times without stretching its wall. Gentleness is the watchword.

Any forceful maneuver increases morbidity. Luminal narrowing or acute angulation may require the operator to retreat judiciously.

Hemorrhage

Hemorrhage during colonoscopy is almost always extrinsic to the colonic lumen. It results from tearing the mesentery or colonic ligaments by vigorously pushing, twisting or pulling the instrument.

Splenic rupture may occur when too much tension is placed on the splenic flexure of the colon, either while advancing the colonoscope or while straightening the splenic flexure.

Vasovagal Reaction

A vasovagal reaction may be recognized when a patient has cold, clammy skin, diaphoresis, bradycardia and hypotension. This reaction occurs when the mesentery and the colon become stretched. It may lead to myocardial infarction or cardiac arrest owing to hypotension and hypovolemia, which result in decreased cardiac output. The patient usually complains of abdominal pain before the onset of the vasovagal reaction. By avoiding a painful procedure, this reaction can be prevented. It is likely that vasovagal reflex occurs more frequently than has been reported.

When this reaction does occur, the endoscopist should terminate the procedure and withdraw the instrument. Insufflated air in the colon should be aspirated on withdrawal of the colonoscope.

If meperidine or a similar analgesic was used as the pre-medication, naloxone (0.4-0.8 mg) should be given intravenously. The patient's legs should be elevated. If hypotension and sweating continue, intravenous fluids and nasal oxygen should be given.

Postcolonoscopy Distention

The so-called postcolonoscopy distention syndrome is characterized by an uncomfortable, painful or distended abdomen after the procedure. A prolonged procedure and excessive insufflation of air are the causes of this syndrome; aspiration of colonic air on withdrawal of the instrument prevents or relieves this syndrome. If the operator fails to reach the cecum after a prolonged attempt, the right side of the abdomen should be compressed gently while insufflated air is being aspirated. This approach may help evacuate air in the right side of the colon.

After colonoscopy, prolonged distention and abdominal pain may be confused with perforation of the bowel. Although these complications are relieved by spontaneous evacuation of air, reinsertion of the colonoscope and aspiration is the treatment of choice. A rectal tube also may be inserted to help evacuate air, if the patient has left the colonoscopy suite.

Roentgenograms of the abdomen help make the diagnosis of excessive distention of the colon. Anticholinergics should not be used during the procedure to prevent this complication.

Volvulus

Volvulus of both the sigmoid colon and the cecum has occurred after colonoscopy. This complication is rare. When the instrument reaches the cecum, any loop that has been made during insertion should be removed before withdrawal of the colonoscope; insufflated air should be aspirated as well.

Infection

Bacterial, viral, parasitic and venereal infections may be transmitted by a colonoscope. It is therefore necessary to sterilize the instrument after examining a patient suspected of having a particular pathogen or transmittable disease (e.g., hepatitis, salmonellosis or amebiasis.) Likewise, patients who are at increased risk for infection, (for example, those who are immunosuppressed and those with leukemia, valvular heart disease or synthetic valves) should be examined with a sterile instrument. They should receive preoperative and postoperative antibiotics by the parenteral route.

Fiberoptic instruments can be sterilized with ethylene oxide, followed by aeration.

Mortality

Reported causes of death associated with colonoscopic procedures include myocardial infarction, pulmonary embolus, respiratory arrest, splenic rupture and sepsis secondary to colonic perforation.

BIOPSY

During procedures involving biopsy, a few cases of perforation have been reported. Careless and rapid introduction of the biopsy forceps against the colonic mucosa, especially in patients with inflammatory bowel disease, may result in perforation of the bowel. The operator or assistant should insert the biopsy forceps only when he or she has a clear and unobstructed view of the operative (visual) field.

Hemorrhage after biopsy is usually negligible. Vascular lesions should not be biopsied.

COLONOSCOPIC POLYPECTOMY

The most likely complications are perforation and hemorrhage. A cautious approach prevents these complications.

Table 13. Colonoscopic Complications in
5,500 Polypectomy Patients

Hemorrhage, hospitalized	24
Blood transfusion	6
Colon resection (one had carcinoma)	2
Perforation, free air	2
Conservative treatment (minimal symptoms)	1
Subphrenic abscess (drained 10 ml of pus)	1
Inability to transect (heavy and short stalk)	2
Transmural burn or diverticulitis (24 hours later fever and localized tenderness)	1

The fear of explosion and the need for carbon dioxide insufflation have been based on misconceptions. We have analyzed colonic gas content in properly prepared bowels and have demonstrated that explosive gases are either absent or present in insignificant amounts. If a colon has not been completely cleansed, the operator should not even attempt polypectomy.

Perforation

Perforation or coagulation of the colon during polypectomy occurs when excess heat is applied to the bowel wall. In our experience with 5,500 patients, only one required operative drainage for a subphrenic abscess two months after a perforation. One patient with a benign perforation was treated conservatively, without sequelae (Table 13).

Over the past several years, we have been queried on many occasions regarding perforation of the colon during colonoscopic polypectomy. The causes of perforation are as follows:

1. Errors in manual technique and poor assessment of polyp structure
   a. Improper application and manipulation of the snare-wire
   b. Uneven return of the tip of the snare-wire into the polyethylene tube
2. Attempting polypectomy with poor visualization
3. Snare-wire breakage and penetration of the bowel
4. Excessive electric current, either because of incorrect dial setting or malfunction of the electrocautery unit

Errors in Technique

In the first example, the snare-wire is applied too close to the base of the stalk. This approach may result in extension of coagulation to the bowel wall (Fig. 272a).

In the second example, the snare-wire is pushed against the bowel wall. The correct approach is to pull the stalk of the polyp toward the center of the lumen of the colon. Slight tenting of the stalk into the lumen is absolutely necessary. A pedunculated polyp should be transected through the neck to assure an adequate margin of safety. Furthermore, when the snare-wire is inadequately placed against the stalk, the proximal part of the snare-wire will coagulate the adjacent bowel wall (Fig. 272b).

In the third example, improper manipulation of the tip may cause the snare-wire to push against the opposite wall, resulting in coagulation and perforation (snare-wire breakage) (Fig. 272c). The snare-wire should be around the center or distal part of the stalk, and the polyp head should lightly touch the opposite wall. Coagulation current flows through the polyp head to the bowel wall, so the small area of conduction between the head of the polyp and the bowel wall concentrates the current at the point of contact. Concentration of current may cause perforation, which can be prevented by oscillating the polyp head gently or by moving either the scope or snare-wire during coagulation (Fig. 272d).

A large sessile polyp may override a mucosal fold. When snaring the base, mucosa may be included in the wire loop, resulting in perforation. This type of polyp is frequently found in the right, or transverse, colon. This error

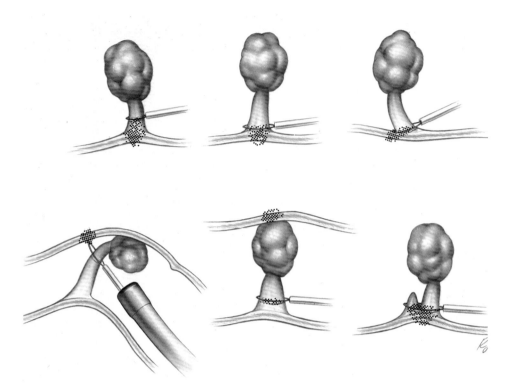

Fig. 272. Perforation of the colon.

a: Prolonged application of excessive coagulation current allows the burn to extend through the stalk to the wall.

b: A snare applied too close to the base of the stalk causes a transmural burn and perforation.

c: If the tip of the snare comes in contact with the adjacent colonic wall, the burn becomes more extensive.

d: If the tip of the snare comes in contact with the opposite wall during excision, it produces a burn and perforation. **c** and **d**

are a result of poor control of the tip of the colonoscope.

e: In theory, a small contact surface between the head of the polyp and the opposite wall may result in extensive coagulation of the opposite wall before a large polyp can be transected completely. This problem can be prevented by oscillating either the catheter or the colonoscope during application of the coagulation current.

f: Inadvertent snaring of adjacent mucosa results in a burn and perforation.

should be avoided by removing the lesion in several segments. A barium enema can be helpful in assessing this type of polyp before the procedure (Fig. 273a).

Prolonged coagulation of the wide base of a large sessile polyp may cause perforation of the bowel wall, which can be avoided by removing the lesion in a piecemeal fashion (Fig. 273b).

Polypoid carcinoma or sessile adenomas with invasive malignant degeneration are usually difficult to transect at the base. The difficulty is caused by the presence of fibrotic tissue within the carcinoma and adjacent tissues. Transec-

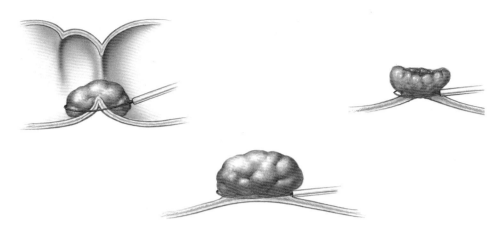

Fig. 273. Perforation.
a: Wide-based, sessile polyp overrides a fold, especially in the right colon. Ensnarement at the base may lead to perforation.
b: With a large, wide-based, sessile polyp, attempts at complete removal at the base may cause perforation.
c: With this puckering polypoid carcinoma, the colonic wall is thinned and fibrosed. Transsection through this area leads to perforation.

tion of such lesions may require more time and increased current, which may result in a transmural burn or perforation. Perforation may occur during transection of a lesion in which malignant cells invade the colonic wall. Puckering of the bowel wall by carcinoma may easily cause perforation when the snare-wire is used to transect the lesion because of thinning of the wall and the prolonged coagulation time required for transection (Fig. 273c).

If a barium enema shows a definite contour defect, the lesion should not be removed endoscopically, even if it is smaller than 1.0 cm.

Before transecting such a lesion, the operator should push or move it with the tip of the colonoscope or the snare-wire. If the lesion cannot be moved without moving colonic mucosa, the tumor is invading into or beyond the submucosa and should not be removed.

Patients who complain of sharp abdominal pain during snare cauterization have incurred a transmural burn. For such patients, application of current should cease immediately. The snare-wire should be removed and the colonoscope should be withdrawn after aspiration of insufflated air. A series of chest and upright abdominal x-ray films should then be taken to rule out free perforation.

When free perforation is obvious to the colonoscopist or when free air is visualized on an x-ray film, prompt operative intervention is required. When laparotomy is carried out for perforation, a histologic report on the excised specimen should be obtained quickly to determine whether bowel resection is necessary. If a patient is treated conservatively and shows progression of signs and symptoms, exploratory laparotomy should be performed.

Hemorrhage

Immediate Hemorrhage

Immediate hemorrhage during polypectomy is caused by inadequate coagulation during transection of the stalk or base of the polyp.

If pulsatile bleeding occurs after transection of the stalk, the operator must be prepared to immediately resnare the stalk with the wire loop. It may be coagulated without attempting to transect the pedicle, or if the stalk is heavy and short, it can be held snugly for a minimum of 15 minutes until it becomes edematous. The operator can then slowly release the loop and, if no further bleeding occurs, the entire snare can be removed.

If bleeding persists, the snare should be tightened again, and the operator may have to wait 15-20 minutes before releasing the snare a second time (Figs. 274 and 275).

If resnaring of the pedicle is not possible, the colonoscope should be withdrawn and the patient closely observed. Since most hemorrhages cease spontaneously, repeated attempts at endoscopic control may be unnecessary and even harmful.

When bleeding cannot be controlled endoscopically, blood should be typed and cross-matched. The patient should be transferred to an intensive care unit for careful observation and restriction of oral intake.

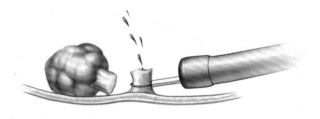

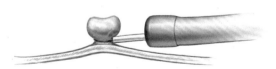

Fig. 274. *Management of pulsatile bleeding.*
a: Pulsatile bleeding may occur immediately after transection of the stalk. The residual stalk must be resnared at once, before blood obscures the operative field.
b: Edema resulting after 15-20 minutes compresses the enclosed blood vessel *and prevents further bleeding. Further coagulation of the cut end of the stalk is contraindicated because 1) hemorrhage cannot be controlled by direct coagulation of the artery; 2) the artery would be further exposed; and 3) normal colonic mucosa that compresses the vessel would be destroyed.*

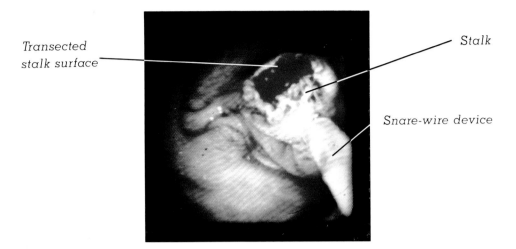

Transected
stalk surface

Stalk

Snare-wire device

Fig. 275. *Endoscopic view of a residual stalk strangulated by a snare-wire. Note the edematous, swollen stalk. No active bleeding is present.*

Delayed Hemorrhage

In rare cases, a patient returns to the hospital emergency room with massive rectal bleeding. Bleeding may occur two to 14 days after polypectomy. This reaction is presumably due to sloughing of the coagulation site.

We have seen 24 such episodes among 5,500 patients (see Table 13). Six of the 24 patients required blood transfusions.

Three of the 24 patients took aspirin (more than 3 tablets/day), and two took an anticoagulant (warfarin or heparin) on the fifth postoperative day.

Eleven patients drank more than 2 ounces of alcohol several hours before the bleeding episode; six patients reported excessive physical exercise, including sit-ups, long walks, jogging, tennis and carrying heavy luggage.

These patients should be hospitalized and vital signs monitored for orthostatic changes. Blood transfusions may be given, if necessary. In our experience, this type of bleeding has been self-limited and usually does not require surgical intervention.

If laparotomy is being considered to control the bleeding, mesenteric angiography should first be done to localize the bleeding site. This is required when numerous polyps in the left and right colon have been excised during one session or when the patient has coexisting diverticular disease.

Transmural Colonic Coagulation

This complication occurs during removal of polyps by prolonged application of electric current to a stalk or base. When transmural coagulation occurs, the patient has abdominal pain, direct and rebound tenderness, low-grade fever and leukocytosis. These signs and symptoms occur six to 12 hours after poly-pectomy.

Free air or retroperitoneal extravasation of air does not accompany this com-plication.

Patients with this complication should be observed in the hospital, receive nothing by mouth, and be given intravenous fluids and broad-spectrum antibi-otics. Spontaneous recovery in two to five days should be anticipated.

Inability to Transect a Stalk

On rare occasions, the operator may be unable to transect a polyp or stalk with the snare-wire. This situation arises when the stalk or the base of the polyp is very thick. Such polyps are frequently too large to be excised with a commer-cial snare device. We have encountered this situation twice and recommend removing the homemade snare-wire in the following way:

1. Make as large a loop as possible with the snare-wire.
2. Slide out the Teflon tubing, removing it entirely from the biopsy channel of the colonoscope.
3. Slowly remove the colonoscope from the patient, leaving behind the snare-wire.
4. Gently pull on the long strand of the snare-wire, thus removing the wire completely. (This procedure can be accomplished only with a homemade hand snare.)

If the snare-wire becomes trapped within the base or the stalk of a polyp, aggressive attempts at resection using a strong coagulation or cutting current may cause perforation of the colon.

With proper technique, sound judgment and experience, the incidence of such complications should be low and the mortality nonexistent. The results of colonoscopic polypectomy are far superior to those previously obtained by transabdominal colotomy and polypectomy, and the cost is far less.

18

Follow-up Examination

As we have previously reported, colonoscopy is much more accurate than a barium enema, particularly for detecting small colonic lesions.

A fiberoptic endoscope, which transmits a clear, magnified image, and which also has biopsy capabilities, should be used for follow-up examinations.

It is impossible to state with certainty the time interval at which a follow-up examination should be done. Nonetheless, I have been impressed by the low incidence of new polyps and metachronous lesions encountered during repeat examinations at six months to one year. I have too few patients to allow statistical analysis, but I intend to continue this policy for repeat examinations until computer analysis of the data is complete.

After Polypectomy

Benign Neoplastic Polyps

For patients in this category, follow-up colonoscopic examinations are done at intervals of 12 to 30 months, depending on the morphologic appearance of the polyp, whether there were many polyps, whether there is a family history of polyps or colonic cancer and the age at which the initial polypectomy was done.

Polyps with Dysplasia or Carcinoma in Situ or Wide-Based Sessile Polyps with Villous Components

Patients in this category receive a first follow-up examination three months after complete removal of the polyp. Reexamination is recommended six months after the first follow-up examination. Thereafter, the examinations are done at 12- to 30-month intervals.

Previous Malignant Tumors of the Colon

The examination schedule for patients who have undergone resection of the colon for carcinoma should be every six months for two years after the procedure and every one to two years thereafter, depending on the age of the patient and the type of procedure performed.

A stool test for occult blood should be done every six months for four years.

Underlying Premalignant Disease of the Colon

Included in this group are patients with inflammatory bowel disease and any of the inherited polyposes. Such patients should undergo barium enema or colonoscopy (or both) at least once a year.

If a colonic stricture is seen in patients with inflammatory bowel disease, the examination should be done every six months and should include biopsy and cytologic smears of the stricture.

Family History of Polyps and Malignant Tumors of the Colon

All such patients should undergo barium enema or colonoscopy (or both) every two to three years if they are over 40 years of age. However, if colonic symptoms (especially rectal bleeding) develop in the intervening period, colonoscopy should be performed regardless of the patient's age. A stool test for occult blood is recommended annually.

Persons Beyond Age 40

Routine examination for asymptomatic patients over age 40 would consist of a stool test for occult blood once a year and a barium enema or colonoscopy (or both) every 30 to 36 months.

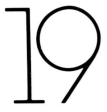

Special Applications of Colonoscopy

This chapter will review special diagnostic and therapeutic applications of colonoscopy, some of which eliminate or reduce the need for exploratory surgery on an elective or emergency basis.

Colonoscopy Via Colostomy

Not infrequently a transverse colostomy is performed for obstruction in the left colon, especially the sigmoid, without a definite diagnosis. After recovery from emergency surgery, the patient undergoes contrast studies to determine the exact nature of the cause of obstruction (Figs. 276 and 277). The results of these

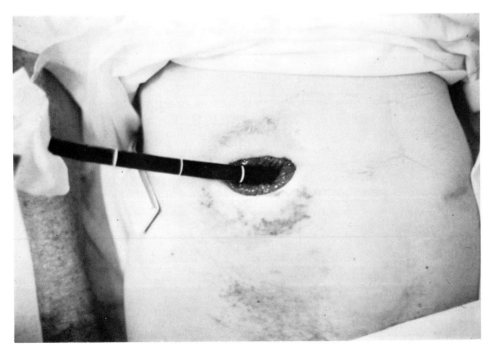

Fig. 276. Colonoscopy being performed via diverting a colostomy stoma. The patient is placed in the supine or right lateral recumbent position.

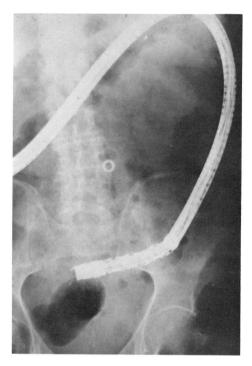

Fig. 277. *X-ray film of the patient shown in Fig. 276. The colonoscope is advanced to the midsigmoid colon, at which point an obstructive lesion is encountered.*

studies are frequently equivocal (i.e., the presence of diverticuli in the sigmoid colon does not guarantee that diverticulitis is the cause of the obstruction). Even clinical signs of fever and left lower quadrant tenderness may accompany a carcinoma that has perforated. For this reason, patients who have had an emergency colostomy for obstruction should undergo colonoscopy from both directions (efferent limb of loop colostomy and rectum) (Fig. 278). In this way, the correct diagnosis usually can be made, including tissue confirmation and plans for subsequent resection made intelligently. It has been our policy as well to examine the afferent limb to the cecum to rule out synchronous disease.

Preparation for endoscopic evaluation via a colostomy is similar to that for routine colonoscopy, as follows:

1. Clear fluids for 24 hours before examination
2. Citrate of magnesia (5-10 ounces) or castor oil (1-2 ounces) the night before
3. Colostomy and rectal irrigation with tap water one to three hours before examination

Examination of such patients begins at the rectum, with the colostomy appliance left in place to seal the stoma; insufflated air pressure thus will be maintained. Even when an examination is performed by an experienced endoscopist with a minimum of insufflation, the presence of the bag prevents fecal soaking of the abdominal wall.

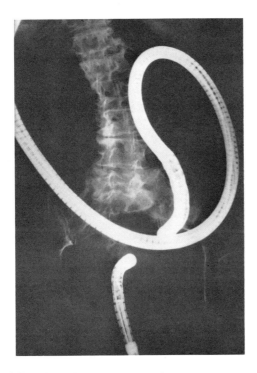

Fig. 278. The obstructive lesion is examined by inserting the colonoscope via the colostomy and rectally. (An obstructing area due to diverticular disease is clearly localized by this method.) Any distal obstruction in a patient with a diverting colostomy may be investigated in this manner.

At the end of the rectal examination, the patient is placed in the supine position. The colonoscope is then introduced into the distal limb, through the colostomy bag, if desired. As noted above, this approach not only maintains insufflated air pressure but also protects the patient against fecal spillage.

Any prolapse of the colostomy must be reduced before the examination to avoid the pressure ischemia that can occur when the colon is compressed between the instrument and the fascial ring. Not only does this approach permit a less traumatic examination, but if air escapes around the instrument, the skin edges around the stoma may be brought together by an assistant to maintain effective insufflation. Both the skin edges and the colostomy mucosa should be well lubricated during the examination.

Colonoscopy via an end-sigmoid colostomy is performed in a manner similar to that described above because there is no need for a rectal examination (unless a Hartmann procedure was done). The patient is first placed in the supine position. The dose of a cathartic may be increased, as in routine colonoscopy.

Endoscopy Via Ileostomy

Examination through an ileostomy may be necessary to evaluate inflammatory bowel disease. The technique is similar to that of an end-colostomy, with certain modifications. Preparation consists of clear fluids only for 24 hours before the examination and ileostomy irrigation with tap water or normal saline one to two hours before the examination. No cathartic should be given. The stoma usually admits only the tip of the little finger, and therefore an instrument 1 cm in diameter or less. Pediatric instruments, such as the Olympus GIF-P2 or GIF-Q, or Pentax FG28A or Fujinon EGD, are usually used. Since these instruments are designed and used for upper endoscopy, ileostomy examination should be performed at the end of the day's schedule, and the instrument should be gas sterilized by the nurse after using it in the bowel.

Internal Colonic Fistula

In patients with suspected internal colonic fistula, colonoscopy can help demonstrate the extent of the fistulous tract and detect the cause of the fistula. Diagnostic colonoscopy is carried out in the usual manner. Identification of a fistulous opening is confirmed by introducing a Teflon catheter through the biopsy channel and into the fistulous opening. Gastrografin is injected and monitored via image intensification. Thus, the entire fistulous tract can be demonstrated. In patients with colocutaneous fistulae, injection of a small amount of colored solution via cutaneous openings can identify the area of colonic opening. Fig. 279 shows a fistulous tract from the sigmoid to the cecum.

Removing Foreign Bodies

Foreign bodies swallowed either accidentally or intentionally often leave the stomach before the patient is seen by a physician. Such objects may become

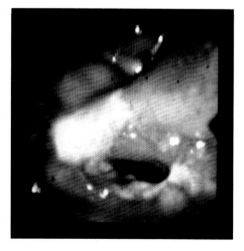

Fig. 279. *Endoscopic view of a fistulous orifice in the cecum.*

trapped in the terminal ileum just proximal to the ileocecal valve. If they fail to pass spontaneously after a reasonable period (one to two weeks) and are not completely obstructing, endoscopic removal should be attempted. Various foreign body forceps or snare-wires can be inserted through the biopsy channel of the colonoscope. Although such devices help mobilize a foreign body out of the terminal ileum and into the cecum, retrieval is usually done with a snare-wire. This snare-wire used should be a homemade type that does not have a handle, so that if the foreign body cannot be removed after the wire is in place, it can be removed by the method described in Chapter 18.

Fig. 280 shows a dental crown in the terminal ileum two weeks after it was swallowed. The colonoscope was introduced into the cecum, and the crown was mobilized with the foreign body forceps and brought into the cecum (Fig. 281). It was then lassoed with a snare-wire and retrieved (Figs. 282 and 283).

Reducing High Sigmoid Volvulus

Sigmoid volvulus is usually treated with sigmoidoscopic reduction and rectal tube placement. If this technique fails, laparotomy and reduction of the volvulus is performed. Before resorting to laparotomy, colonoscopy should be attempted. In some cases, the colonoscope can be inserted into the distended segment, and decompression will take place around the instrument. Quick reflexes on the part of the endoscopist are sometimes necessary.

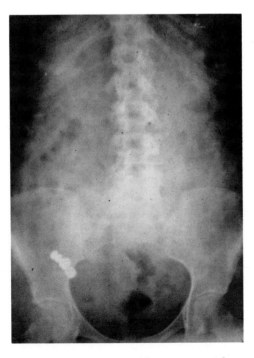

Fig. 280. A 26-year-old woman with a gold dental crown in the distal terminal ileum. It was accidentally swallowed 3 weeks before the examination.

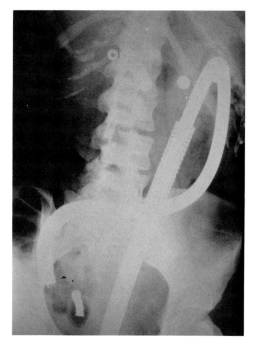

Fig. 281. Colonoscope introduced to the terminal ileum. The foreign body was trapped just above the ileocecal valve. It was mobilized into the cecum using a foreign body forceps, then ensnared with a snare-wire.

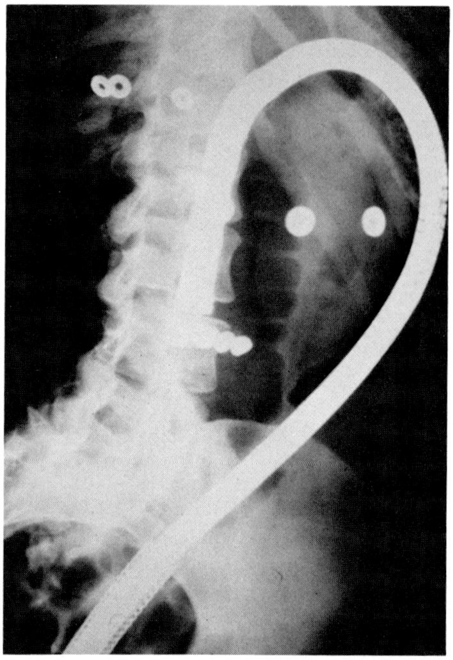

Fig. 282. A gold dental crown being removed by a snare-wire inserted endoscopically. X-ray film was taken with the foreign body mobilized to the mid-transverse colon.

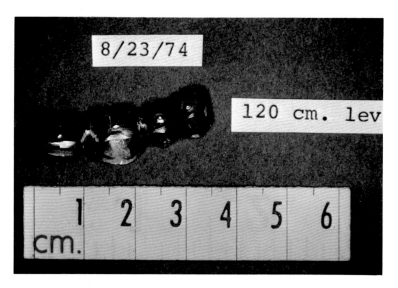

Fig. 283. Dental crown removed endoscopically.

Reducing Intussusception

Colocolonic intussusception caused by large benign polyps may be reduced endoscopically. Reduction is accomplished by gently "nudging" the head of the intussusception back with the tip of the colonscope and with air insufflation until the procedure is complete. This technique usually does not work for colonic carcinoma.

Ileocolic intussusception can, in theory, be managed in the same manner if barium enema reduction is unsuccessful. No such cases have been reported, and I have not had experience with this entity.

Fig. 284 shows a large polypoid lesion of the right transverse colon. During preparation for colonoscopic polypectomy, the patient complained of crampy abdominal pain and passed some blood. At colonoscopy, the polypoid lesion that had previously been seen in the right transverse colon was now occluding the lumen of the sigmoid colon at 30 cm. The intussusception was reduced by pushing the tumor back with the tip of the instrument. Partial excision of the lesion was performed. The excised specimens revealed infiltrating adenocarcinoma, and the patient underwent colonic resection.

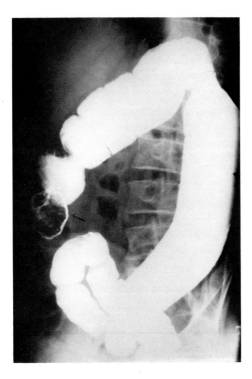

Fig. 284. A large villous adenoma of the ascending colon causing mechanical obstruction secondary to intussusception. The intussusception was reduced by the colonoscope, and the lesion was excised endoscopically.

Bibliography

A Guide to Chemical Disinfection and Sterilization for Hospitals and Related Care Facilities. Michigan Department of Health, 1963.

Adler VG, Mitchell JP: The disinfection of heat sensitive surgical instruments, in Shapton DA, Board RG (eds): *Safety in Microbiology*. London, Academic Press, 1972.

Almy TP: Diverticular disease of the colon—the new look. *Gastroenterology* 49:109, 1965.

Altmeier WA, Culbertson WR, Hummel RP: Surgical considerations of endogenous infections—sources, types and methods of control. *Surg Clin Am* 48:227, 1968.

Arullani A, Paoluzzi P, Capurso L: Endoscopy of the colon, in *Proceedings of the 1st European Congress on Digestive Endoscopy*, Prague, 1968, pp 2-6.

Axon ATR, Cotton PB, Phillips I, et al: Disinfection of gastrointestinal fibre endoscopes. *Lancet* 656, April 1974.

Axtell LM, Chiazzo L Jr: Changing relative frequency of cancers of the colon and rectum in the U.S. *Cancer* 19:750, 1966.

Bacon HE, Holoman MB, Chinprahast K: Pancoloniscopy: Is it a valuable procedure? *Dis Colon Rectum* 6:311, 1963.

Banche M, Rossini FP, Ferrari A, et al: The role of colonoscopy in the differential diagnosis between idiopathic ulcerative colitis and Crohn's disease of the colon. 39th Annual Convention, American College of Gastroenterology, Florida, October 1974.

Banez AV: Operative fiberoptic colonoscopy. Personal communication, 1973.

Bartelheimer W, Remmele W, Otteniann R: Colonoscopic recognition of hemangiomas in the colon ascendens. Case report of so-called cryptogenic gastrointestinal bleeding. *Endoscopy* 4:100, 1972.

Becker GL, Prevention of gas explosions in the large bowel during electrosurgery. *Surg Gynecol Obstet* 97:463, 1953.

Becker H, Schuelke K: Koloskopie—Ein Verfahrren zur intraoperativen Endoskopischen Tumordiagnostik des Dickdarms. *Endoscopy* 3:182, 1970.

Beecham HJ III, Cohen ML, Parkin WE: Salmonella typhimurium transmission by fiberoptic upper gastrointestinal endoscopy. *J Am Med Ass* 241:1013, 1979.

Bennett JA, Salmon PR, Branch RA, et al: The use of inhalational anaesthesia during fibre-optic colonoscopy. *Anaesthesia* 26:294, 1971.

Berci G, Panish JF, Schapiro M, et al: Complications of colonoscopy and polypectomy. *Gastroenterology* 67:584, 1974.

Berezov YE, Sotnikov VN, Kornilov YM: Colonoscopy in diagnosing disease of the large intestine (in Russian). *Vestn Akad Med Nauk SSR* 27(2):65, 1972.

Berman PM, Kirsner JB: Current knowledge of diverticular disease of the colon. *Am J Dig Dis* 17:741, 1972.

Berry LH: *Gastrointestinal Pan-endoscopy*. Springfield, Ill, Charles C Thomas, Publisher, 1974.

Bloom BS, Goldhaber SZ, Sugarbaker PH, et al: Fiberoptics: Morbidity and cost. *N Engl J Med* 288:368, 1973.

Bockus HL: *Gastroenterology*, Vol. II. Philadelphia, WB Saunders, 1976.

Bognel JC, Liguory A, Bitoun A, et al: L'exerese des polypes par coloscopie. Vie Medicale 36, 4615-4626-Novembre 1973.

Bolt RJ: Sigmoidoscopy in detection and diagnosis in the asymptomatic individual. *Cancer (Philadelphia)* 28:121, 1971.

Bond WW, Moncada RE: Viral hepatitis B infection risk in flexible fiberoptic endoscopy. *Gastrointest Endosc* 24:225, 1978.

Bruch CW: Gaseous sterilization. *Annu Rev Microbiol* 15:245, 1961.

Bruwer A, Bargen JA, Kierland RR: Surface pigmentation and generalized intestinal polyposis (Peutz-Jeghers syndrome). *Mayo Clin Proc* 29:168, 1954.

Burdick D, Prior JT, Scanlon GT: Peutz-Jeghers syndrome: A clinical-pathological study of a large family with a ten year follow-up. *Cancer (Philadelphia)* 16:854, 1963.

Bussey H Jr, Wallace MH, Morson BC: Metachronous carcinoma of the large intestine and intestinal polyps. *Proc R Soc Med* 60:208, 1967.

Casarella WJ, Galloway SJ, Taxin RN, et al: "Lower" gastrointestinal tract hemorrhage: New concepts based on arteriography. *Am J Radiol* 121:357, 1974.

Carroll KJ: Unusual explosion during electrosurgery. *Br Med J* 2:117, 1964.

Carter HG: Explosion in the colon during electrodesiccation of polyps. *Am J Surg* 84:514, 1952.

Cavenach AJM, Rintoul RF: Cancer of the bowel. *Br Med J* 3:165, 1972.

Chabanon R: La polypectomie coloscopique. *Acta Gastro-enterol Belg* 37:166, 1974.

Chang FM, Sakai Y, Ashizawa S: Bacterial pollution and disinfection of the colonofiberscope. 1. An investigation of traditional sterilization methods. *Dig Dis* 18(11) 1973.

Chang FM, Sakai Y, Ashizawa S: Bacterial pollution and disinfection of the colonfiberscope. 2. Ethylene oxide gas sterilization. *Dig Dis* 18:951, 1973.

Christie J, Shinya H: Indications for fiberoptic colonoscopy. *South Med J* 68(7):881, 1975.

Christie J: Fiberoptic colonoscopy: Diagnostic value in 250 consecutive patients. *South Med J* 69:540, 1976.

Christie J: Colonoscopic excision of sessile polyps. *Am J Gastroenterol* 66:23, 1976.

Christie J: Colonoscopic excision of large sessile polyps. *Am J Gastroenterol* 67:430, 1977.

Christie J: Colonoscopic removal of sessile colonic lesions. *Dis Colon Rectum* 21:11, 1978.

Classen M, Fruhmorgen P, Koch H, et al: Peroral enteroscopy of the small and the large intestine. *Endoscopy* 4:157, 1972.

Classen M, Koch H, Fruhmorgen P: Perorale enteroskiopie. *Med Trib* 3:47a, 1971.

Colcher H: Colonoscopie, quo vadis. *Ann Gastroenterol Hepat* 7:247, 1971.

Colcher H: Progress in gastrointestinal endoscopic instrumentation in the past decade. *Gastrointest Endosc* 17:169, 1971.

Colcock BP: *Diverticular Disease of the Colon*. Philadelphia, WB Saunders, 1971, pp 125-128.

Colcock BP: Surgical treatment of diverticulitis—twenty years' experience. *Am J Surg* 115:264, 1968.

Connell AM: Dietary fiber and diverticular disease. *Hosp Pract* 11:3, 1976.

Cornet A, Barbier JP, Carayon P, et al: Polypes coliques. Interet du depistage et de l'identification par la coloscopie. *Arch Fr Mal Appar Dig* 60:261, 1971.

Cotton PB, Williams CB: Fibreoptic instruments for gastrointestinal endoscopy. *Br J Hosp Med* 8:35, 1972.

Crespon B, Housset P, Campora A, et al: Apport de la colonoscopie d'urgence dans les hemorrhagies digestives basses. *Acta Endosc Radiocinematogr* III (5):133, 1973.

Crumpacker EL, Baker SP: Proctosigmoidoscopy in periodic health examinations. *J Am Med Ass* 78:1033, 1961.

Culp, CE: New studies of the eolonic polyp and cancer. *Surg Clin N Am* 47:955, 1967.

Curtiss LE: High frequency currents in endoscopy: A review of principles and precautions. *Gastrointest Endosc,* 1973.

Dean ACB: Problems with coloscopic polypectomy. *Endoscopy* 5:121, 1973.

Dean ACB: Coloscopy in diagnostic problems in the large bowel. *Acta gastro-enterol Belg* 37:145, 1973.

Dean ACB, Newell JP: Colonoscopy in the differential diagnosis of carcinoma from diverticulitis of the sigmoid colon. *Br J Surg,* 1973.

Dean ACB, Shearman DJC: A clinical evaluation of the Olympus CF-SB fibreoptic colonoscope, in *Proceedings of the IInd World Congress of Gastrointestinal Endoscopy,* Rome-Copenhagen, 1970.

DeBeer R, Geffen A, Ozoktay S, et al: Comparison of colonoscopy and contrast x-ray study in diagnosis of colorectal disease. *JAOA* 75:569, 1976.

Deddish MR, Hertz RE: Colotomy and coloscopy in the management of neoplasm of the colon. *Dis Colon Rectum* 2:133, 1959.

De La Santa Lopez J, et al: Fibrocolonoscopia: technica y valoracion clinica. *Rev Esp Enferm Apar Dis* 39:651, 1973.

Devrode GJ, Taylor WF, Sauer WG, et al: Cancer risk and life expectancy of children with ulcerative colitis. *N Engl J Med* 285:17, 1971.

Deyhle P: Technik und klinische bedeutung. Endoskopiekongress, Deutsche Gesellschaft tuer Endoskopie, Erlangen, 1971.

Deyhle P: Flexible steel wire for the maintenance of the straightening of the sigmoid and transverse colon during coloscopy. *Endoscopy* 4:36, 1972.

Deyhle P: A plastic tube for the maintenance of the straightening of the sigmoid colon during colonoscopy. *Endoscopy* 4:224, 1972.

Deyhle P, Demling L: Coloscopy—technique; results, indication. *Endoscopy* 3:143, 1971.

Deyhle P, Jenny S, Fumagalli I: Endoskopische Polypectomie in proximalen Kolon. *Dtsch Med Wochenschr* 98:219, 1973.

Deyhle P, Ottenjann R: Zur transintestinalen intubation, in Ottenjann R (ed): *Fortschritte der Endoskopie,* ed 2. Stuttgart, Schattauer, 1970.

Dilawari JB, Parkinson C, Riddel RH, et al: Colonoscopy in the investigation of ulcerative colitis (Abstr). *Gut* 14:426, 1973.

Dive C, Vanheuverzwijn R: Aspects endoscopiques de la colite granulomateuse. *Acta Gastro-enterol Belg* 37:150, 1974.

Doos WG, Wolff WI, Shinya H, et al: Carcinoembryonic antigen levels in patients with colorectal polyps. *Cancer (Philadelphia)* 36:1196, 1975.

Dunphy JE: In discussion of paper by Wolff and Shinya. *Ann Surg* 178:377, 1973.

Eddy HJ: Intracolonic electro-snare polypectomy using flexible fiberoptic colonoscopes, in *Communicationes 2e Congres Europeen d'Endoscopie Digestive,* Paris, 1972.

Eddy JH, Finnerty UR: Case report: Multiple Undiagnosed Polyps found during Colonoscopy on a Three Year Old Child, in *Communicationes 2e Congres Europeen d'Endoscopie Digestive,* Paris, 1972.

Enterline HT: Management of polypoid lesions. *J Am Med Ass* 231:967, 1975.

Espiner H, Salmon PR, Teague R, et al: Operative colonoscopy. *Br Med J* 1:453, 1973.

Ewe K: Endoskopie des Rektums und Kolons. *Therapiewoche* 19:567, 1969.

Faggioli F, Mattei M: La colonoscopia. *Gazz Sanit* :94, 1972.

Fenoglio CM, Kane GI, Lane N: Distribution of human colonic lymphatics in normal hyperplastic and adenomatous tissue. *Gastroenterology* 64:51, 1972.

Fenoglio CM, Lane N: The anatomic precursor of colorectal cancer. *Cancer (Philadelphia)* 34:819, 1974.

Fiorini E, Fratton A, Polettini FL, et al: Contribution to the endoscopic study of the left colon, in *Proceedings of the IInd World Congress of Gastrointestinal Endoscopy*, Rome-Copenhagen, 1970.

Fitts WT Jr: Adenomas of the colon and rectum. *Am J Surg* 101:87, 1961.

Forde KA: Colonoscopy in complicated diverticular disease. *Gastrointest Endosc* 23:192, 1977.

Fox JA: Mucosal biopsy of the colon by retrograde intubation. Results and applications. *Br J Surg* 54:867, 1967.

Fox JA: Technik der retrograden Kolonsondierung und hohen Kolonbiopsie, in *Fortschritte der Endoskopie*, ed 1. Stuttgart, Schattauer, 1969.

Fox JA: Retrograde colonoscopy. *Endoscopy* 4:182, 1969.

Fox JA, Kriel L: Technique of retrograde colonic intubation and its initial application to high colonic biopsy. *Gut* 8:77, 1967.

Fox MJA: Maladie de Crohn. Colonoscopie. *Arch Fr Mal Appar Dig* 61(4-5):373, 1972.

Francillon J, Vignal J, Lesbros F, et al: Incidences de la colonoscopie et de l'anatomie pathologique sur la tactique chirurgicale concernant les polypes due colon et du rectum. *Chirurgie* 97:322, 1971.

Frient WG: Colonoscopy and polypectomy. *Northwest Med* 71:613, 1972.

Frotz H, Gheorghiu T: Endoscopic diagnosis of colonic diseases. *Leber Magen Darm* 3:124, 1973.

Frotz H, Gheorghiu T, Philippen R: Koloscopie mit fiberoptischen Instrumenten. *Med Welt* 23:193, 1972.

Fruhmorgen P: Diagnosis of inflammatory diseases of the colon by coloscopy. *Acta Gastro-enterol Belg* 37:154, 1974.

Gabriellsson N, Grandquist S, Ohlsen H: Colonoscopy: Technique, indications, and results. *Lakartidningen* 69/39 4377, 1972.

Gabriellsson N, Grandquist S, Ohlsen H: Colonoscopy with the aid of a steel wire to stiffen the fiberscope. *Endoscopy* 4:217, 1972.

Gaisford WD: Gastrointestinal polypectomy via the fiberendoscope. *Arch Surg* 106:453, 1973.

Gaisford WD: Gastrointestinal fiberendoscopy. *Am J Surg* 124:744, 1972.

Gaisford WD: Fiberendoscopy of the cecum and terminal ileum. *Gastrointest Endosc* 21:13, 1974.

Gangarosa EJ, Beisel WR: A simple technic for colonic biopsy of the rectum. *Gastroenterology* 42:157, 1962.

Ghazi A, Shinya H, Wolff WI: Treatment of volvulus of the colon by colonoscopy. *Ann Surg* 183:263, 1976.

Gilbertsen VA: Proctosigmoidoscopy and polypectomy in reducing the incidence of rectal cancer. *Cancer (Philadelphia)* 34:936, 1974.

Gilbertsen VA, Knatternd GI, Lober PH, et al: Invasive carcinoma of the large intestine—a preventable disease? *Surgery* 57:363, 1965.

Glotzer DJ, Gardner RC, Goldman H, et al: Comparative features and course of ulcerative and granulomatous colitis. *N Engl J Med* 282:582, 1970.

Goldgraber MD, Kirsner JB: Polyps and carcinoma of the colon. *Arch Intern Med* 100:669, 1957.

Golligher JC, Graham ME, DeDombrae FT: Anastomotic dehiscence after anterior resection of rectum. *Br J Surg* 560-692, 1969.

Goodman ML, Gottlieb LS, Zamcheck N: Granular cell myoblastoma of the stomach and colon. *Am J Dig Dis* 7:432, 1962.

Granquist S, Gabriellsson N, Ohlsen H: Colofiberskopie, TV genomlysning, Sam Komplement till rontgenundersohnung. *Abstr Med Rickstamman*, 1971.

Gregg JA, Garabedian M: Colonoscopy. *Surg Clin N Am* 51:661, 1971.

Grinnell RS, Lane N: Benign and malignant adenomatous polyps and papillary adenomas of colon and rectum. *Int Abstr Surg* 106:519, 1958.

Hagihara PF, Parker JC, Griffen WO Jr: Spontaneous ischemic colitis. *Dis Colon Rectum* 20(3):236, 1977.

Harmon ML: Nurses' role in lower gastrointestinal endoscopy. *Surg Clin N Am* 52:1025, 1972.

Hayashi M, Yukama E, Yukama K: Radiology compared with endoscopy for the diagnosis of the cancer of large intestine, in *Communicationes 2e Congres Europeen d'Endoscopie Digestive*, Paris, 1972.

Hedberg S, Schrock S, Sugarbarker P: Cited in discussion of Wolff and Shinya's presentation. *Ann Surg* 178:377, 1973.

Hedrick E: Cleaning and disinfection of flexible fiberoptic endoscopy (FFE) used in gastrointestinal endoscopy. *APIC* December 1978.

Hiratsuka H: Fibercolonoscopy in the diagnostic intestinal string derivation. Method and clinical report on ileocecal observation, in *IInd World Congress of Gastrointestinal Endoscopy*, Rome-Copenhagen, 1970.

Hirshowitz BI, Curtis LE, Peters CW, et al: Demonstration of a new gastroscope—the fiberscope. *Gastroenterology* 35:50, 1958.

Hogan WJ, Stewart ET, Geenen JE, et al: A prospective comparison of the accuracy of colonoscopy vs. air-barium contrast examination for detection of colonic polypoid lesions. Meeting of the American Society for Gastrointestinal Endoscopy, Toronto, May 1977.

Hradsky M, Stockbruegger R, Wennerholm M: Erfahrungen mit der Fibercolonoskopischen Untersuchungamethode bei einem Material von 100 Patienten, in *Communicationes 2e Congres Europeen d'Endoscopie Digestive*, Paris, 1972.

Humphries AI Jr, Shepherd MH, Peters HJ: Peutz-Jeghers syndrome with colonic adenocarcinoma and ovarian tumor. *J Am Med Ass* 197:296, 1966.

Ingelfinger FJ: Malignant potential of colonic polyps, in Ingelfinger FJ, et al (eds): *Controversy in Internal Medicine II*. Philadelphia, WB Saunders, 1974.

Kanazawa T, Tanaka M: Endoscopy of colon. *Gastroenterol Endosc (Tokyo)* 7:398, 1965.

Kaneko M: On pedunculated adenomatous polyps of the colon and rectum with particular reference to their malignant potential. *Mt Sinai J Med NY* 39:112, 1972.

Kansen KK: Coloscopy: An analysis of 120 cases with special regards to the technique. *Endoscopy* 5(2):77, 1973.

Kelly HA: Instruments for use through cylindrical rectal specula, with the patient in the knee-chest position. *Ann Surg* 37:924, 1903.

Kleinfeld G, Gump FR: Complications of colotomy and polypectomy. *Surg Gynecol Obstet* III:726, 1960.

Kobayshi S, Mizuno H, Kasugai T: Early colonic cancer presenting as a pedunculated polyp: Application of fibercolonoscopy for its detection. *Gastrointest Endosc* 20:118, 1974.

Kratzer GL: Colonoscopy—current status. *Dis Colon Rectum* 7:45, 1964.

Kuld HL: Colonoscopy: An examination of the diagnostical efficiency of the long colonoscope, in *Communicationes 2e Congres Europeen d'Endoscopie Digestive*, Paris, 1972.

Kurzon RM, Ortega R, Rywlin AM: The significance of papillary features in polyps of the large intestine. *Am J Clin Pathol* 62:447, 1974.

Lambert R, Moulinier B: La gastro-enterologie a l'ere de l'endoscopie. *Presse Med* 79:939, 1971.

LeFrock JL, Ellis CA, Turchik JB, et al: Transient bacteremia associated with sigmoidoscopy. *N Engl J Med* 289:467, 1973.

Levinson JD, Wall AJ, Kirsner JB: The problem of carcinoma in inflammatory disease of the bowel: Selective case experiences. *South Med J* 65:209, 1972.

Levitt MD, Ingelfinger FJ: Hydrogen and methane production in man. *Ann NY Acad Sci* 150:75, 1968.

Levy AG, Benson JW, Hewlett EL, et al: Saline lavage: A rapid, effective and acceptable method for cleansing the gastrointestinal tract. *Gastrointest Endosc* 24:24, 1977.

Lezak MB, Goldhammer M: Retroperitoneal emphysema after colonoscopy. *Gastroenterology* 66:118, 1974.

Lock MR, Cairns DW, Ritchie JK, et al: The treatment of early colorectal cancer by local excision. *Br J Surg* 65:346, 1978.

Marcozzi G, Montori A: Endoscopy during operation: New diagnostic possibilities, preliminary report. *Chir Gastroenterol* 6:24, 1972.

Margulis AR, Burhenne HJ (eds): *Alimentary Tract Roentgenology*, ed 2. St Louis, CV Mosby, 1973, vol 2.

Marino AWM Jr: Complications of colonoscopy. *Dis Colon Rectum* 1:1, 1978.

Marks, G, Moses ML: The clinical application of flexible fiberoptic colonoscopy. *Surg Clin N Am* 53(3): 1973.

Marshak RH, Janowitz HD, Present DH: Granulomatous colitis in association with diverticula. *N Engl J Med* 283:1080, 1970.

Marston A, Pheils MT, Thomas ML, et al: Ischaemic colitis. *Gut* 7:1, 1966.

Martel W, Robins JM: The barium enema; technique, value and limitations. *Cancer (Philadelphia)* 28:137, 1971.

Matsunaga F, Diot J: The clinical value of sigmoidocamera, in *Proceedings Hedrologicum Collegium*, 83-85, 1965.

Matsunaga F: Colonofiberoscopy, in *Proceedings of the IInd World Congress of Gastrointestinal Endoscopy*, Rome-Copenhagen, 1970.

Matsunaga F, Tajima T: Sigmoidocamera and colonofiberoscope (Japanese). *Geka Shinryo* II:427, 1969.

Matsunaga F, Tajima T: Recent advance in colonofiberscopy, in *Communicationes 2e Congres Europeen d'Endoscopie Digestive*, Paris, 1972.

Matsunaga F, Tajima T, Toda S: The limits of colonofiberscopy in early diagnosis of malignant and inflammatory changes, in *Proceedings of the IInd World Congress of Gastrointestinal Endoscopy*, Rome-Copenhagen, 1970.

Matsunaga F, Tajima T, Toda S, et al: Endoscopic examination of the large bowel. *Sogo Rinsho* 19:325, 1970.

Matsunaga F, Tsushima H, Kuboto T: Photography of the colon. *Gastrointest Endosc* 1:58, 1959.

McSherry CK, Cornell GN, Glenn F: Carcinoma of the colon and rectum. *Ann Surg* 169:502, 1969.

Meyers DS: Colonoscopy (letter). *N Engl J Med* 288:974, 1973.

Montori A, Martinelli V, Viceconte G: Indicazioni e tecnica della pancolonscopia nei soggetti anziani. *Il Prog Med* 30:252, 1974.

Moore AE: Traction sigmoidoscopy. *Surg Clin N Am* 37:1283, 1957.

Moore FD: In discussion of paper by Wolff and Shinya. *Ann Surg* 178:376, 1973.

Mori K, Shinya H, Kalisman M: A composite tumor in tubulovillous adenomas of rectum. *Dis Colon Rectum* 21:7, 1978.

Morrissey JF: Gastrointestinal endoscopy. *Gastroenterology* 62:1241, 1972.

Morson BC: Evolution of cancer of the colon and rectum. *Cancer (Philadelphia)* 34:845, 1974.

Morson BC: Pathology of diverticular disease of the colon. *Clin Gastroenterol* 4:37, 1975.

Morson BC, Bussey HJ: Predisposing causes of intestinal cancer. *Curr Prob Surg* p 81, 1970.

Morson BC, Bussey HJR, Samoorian S: Policy of local excision for early cancer of the colorectum. *Gut* 18:1045, 1977.

Morson BC, Dawson IMP: *Gastrointestinal Pathology.* Oxford, Blackwell Scientific Publications, 1972, p 560.

Myren J, Petersen H: Sigmoido-colonoscopy in out-patients. *Scand J Gastroenterol* 7(Suppl 9):39, 1972.

Nagasako K, Endo M, Takemoto T, et al: The insertion of fibercolonoscope into the cecum and the direct observation of the ileocecal valve. *Endoscopy* 2:123, 1970.

Nagasako K, Nagai K, Suzukih, et al: Fiberscopic diagnosis of early cancer of the colon. *Endoscopy* 4:1, 1972.

Nagasako K, Takemoto T: Fibercolonoscopy without the help of fluoroscopy. *Endoscopy* 4:208, 1972.

Nagasako K, Yazawa C, Takemoto T: Observation of the terminal ileum. *Endoscopy* 1:45, 1971.

Nagy GS: Fibrecolonoscopy. *Med J Aust* 1:378, 1973.

Nedbal J: The diagnostic value of fibrosigmoidoscopy. *Czech Cs Gastroent Vyziva* 27:467, 1973.

Nivatvongs S, Goldberg SM: Management of patients who have polyps containing invasive carcinoma removed via the colonoscope. *Dis Colon Rectum* 21:8, 1978.

Niwa H: On photography of the colon and pharynx using gastrocamera. *Gastrointest Endosc* 2:77, 1960.

Niwa H: Endoscopy of the colon. *Gastroenterol Endosc (Tokyo)* 7:403, 1965.

Niwa H: Clinical study of colonfiberscope. *Gastroenterol Endosc (Tokyo)* II:173, 1969.

Niwa H, Fujino M, Utsumi Y, et al: Clinical experience of colonic fiberscope. *Gastroenterol Endosc (Tokyo)* II:163, 1969.

Ogoshi K, Hara Y, Ashizawa S: New technic for small intestinal fiberoscopy. *Gastrointest Endosc* 20:64, 1973.

Olsen WR: Hemorrhage from diverticular disease of the colon. *Am J Surg* 115:247, 1968.

Oshiba S, Watanabe A: Endoscopy of the colon. *Gastroenterol Endosc (Tokyo)* 7:400, 1965.

Ottenjann R: Colonic polyps and colonoscopic polypectomy. *Endoscopy* 4:212, 1972.

Ottenjann R: Endoskopie und Biopsia des Colon. *Dtsch Med Wochenschr* 28:1372, 1968.

Ottenjann R, Gruner HJ, Bartelheimer W: Fibrocolonoscopia parziale ambulatoriale (fibrosigmoidoscopia). *Minerva Med* 63(93):5233, 1972 (Translation in *Dtsch Med Wochenschr* 97:734, 1972).

Overholt BF: Clinical experience with the fibersigmoidoscope. *Gastrointest Endosc* 15:27, 1968.

Overholt BF: Flexible fiberoptic sigmoidoscope. *Ca* 19:81, 1969.

Overholt BF: Technique of flexible fibersigmoidoscopy. *South Med J* 63:787, 1970.

Overholt BF: Flexible fiberoptic sigmoidoscopy. *Cancer (Philadelphia)* 28:123, 1971.

Painter NS, Burkitt DP: Diverticular disease of the colon: A deficiency disease of Western civilization. *Br Med J* 2:450, 1971.

Panish J, Berci G: Colonoscopy and polypectomy, in *Surgery Annual 1973*. New York, Appleton-Century-Crofts, 1973, pp 211-214.

Paoluzzi P: Total colonoscopy by a "monorail" method, in *Proceedings of the IInd World Congress of Gastrointestinal Endoscopy*, Rome-Copenhagen, 1970.

Pappi JP, Haubrich WS: Endoscopic removal of colon lipomas. *Gastrointest Endosc* 20:66, 1973.

Parks TG: Natural history of diverticular disease of the colon: A review of 521 cases. *Br Med J* 4:639, 1969.

Peutz JLA: Over een zeer merkwaardige, gecombineerde familiaire polyposis van de slijmvliezen van den tractus intestinalis met die vande neutskeelholts en gepaard met eigenaardige pigmentaties can huid-en slijmvliezen. *Ned Maandschr Geneeskd* 10:134, 1921.

Phillips CB, Warshowsky B: Chemical disinfection. *Annu Rev Microbiol* 12:525, 1958.

Polk HC, Spratt JS Jr, Butcher HR: Frequency of multiple primary malignant neoplasms associated with colorectal carcinoma. *Am J Surg* 109:71, 1965.

Ponka JL, Brush BE, Fox JD: Differential diagnosis of carcinoma of the sigmoid and diverticulitis. *J Am Med Ass* 172:515, 1960.

Provenzale L, Revignas A: An original method for guided intubation of the colon. *Gastrointest Endosc* 16:11, 1969.

Ragins H, Shinya H: The explosive potential of colonic gas during colonoscopic electrosurgical polypectomy. *Surg Gynecol Obstet* 138:554, 1974.

Rider JA, Kirsner JB, Mueller HC, et al: Polyps of the colon and rectum. *J Am Med Ass* 170:633, 1959.

Rhodes JB, Zarvgulis JE, Williams CH, et al: Oral electrolyte overload to cleanse the colon for colonoscopy. *Gastrointest Endosc* 24:24, 1977.

Rogers BHG: The safety of carbon dioxide insufflation during colonoscopy. *Gastrointest Endosc* 20:115, 1974.

Rogers BHG, Silvis SE, Nebel OT, et al: Complications of flexible fiberoptic colonoscopy and polypectomy. *Gastrointest Endosc* 22:2, 1975.

Rossini FP, Bonardi L: Diagnosi colonscopica nei confronti delle altre metodiche di diagnosi precose dei tumori del colon. *Minerva Gastroenterol* 19(1):24, 1973.

Sakai Y: Further progress in colonoscopy. *Gastrointest Endosc* 20:143, 1974.

Sakai Y: The technic of colonofiberscopy. *Dis Colon Rectum* 15:403, 1972.

Sakai Y, Ashizawa S: Fiberscopic examination of the rectum and sigmoid colon. *Gastroenterol Lap* 5:281, 1970.

Salmon PR, Branch RA, Collins C, et al: Clinical evaluation of fiberoptic sigmoidoscopy employing the Olympus CF-SB colonoscope. *Gut* 51:729, 1971.

Salmon PR, Teague R, Read AE: Fibre-optic examination of the large bowel: Clinical results in 200 cases, in *Communicationes 2e Congres Europeen d'Endoscopie Digestive*, Paris, 1972.

Sanders CV, Luby JP, Johanson WG, et al: Serratia marcescens infections from inhalation therapy medications: Noscomial outbreak. *Ann Intern Med* 73:15, 1970.

Schulke K, Ungeheuer E: Die coloskopie, eine Methode der intraoperativen Endoskopischen untersuchung des Kolons. *Langenbecks Arch Klin Chir* 322:780, 1968.

Seamen WB: Disease of the colon: New concepts, old problems. Annual oration in memory of Charles M. Gray, M.D., 1905-1969. *Radiology* 100:249, 1971.

Segal S, Diot J, Maffioli C, et al: La coloscopie trans-anale. *Maroc Med* 54:283, 1971.

Seifert E: A new flexible forceps for the removal of polyps from the gastrointestinal tract after successful endoscopic polypectomy. *Endoscopy* 4:226, 1972.

Shatney CH, Lober PH, Gilbertsen V, et al: Management of focally malignant pedunculated adenomatous colorectal polyps. *Dis Colon Rectum* 19:334, 1976.

Shatney HC, Lober PH, Gilbertsen VA, et al: The treatment of pedunculated adenomatous colorectal polyps with focal cancer. *Surg Gynecol Obstet* 139:845, 1974.

Shearman DJC: Colonoscopy in ulcerative colitis. *Scand J Gastroenterol* 8:289, 1973.

Shinya H, Wolff WI: Removal of colonic polyps by fiberoptic colonoscopy. *N Engl J Med* 288:329, 1973.

Shinya H, Wolff WI: Fiberoptic endoscopy of the entire small and large intestine, in *Communicationes 2e Congress Europeen d'Endoscopie Digestive*, Paris, 1972.

Shinya H, Wolff WI: Therapeutic applications of colonfiberoscopy: Polypectomy via the colonfiberscope. *Gastroenterology* 60:830, 1971.

Shinya H, Wolff WI: Therapeutic applications of colonfiberoscopy: Polypectomy via the colonoscope, in *Communications 2e Congres Europeen d'Endoscopie Digestive*, Paris, 1972.

Shinya H, Wolff WI: Colonoscopy, technique, diagnosis and treatment of colonic disease. *Adv Surg* 1975.

Shinya H, Wolff WI: Colonscopic polypectomy: Technique and Safety. *Hosp Pract* September 1975.

Shinya H, Wolff WI: Flexible colonoscopy. *Cancer (Philadelphia)* 37:462, 1976.

Shinya H, Wolff WI: Colonfiberoscopy, in Nyhus LM (ed): *Surgery Annual*. New York, Appleton-Century-Crofts, 1976, vol 8.

Shinya H, Wolff WI: Morphology, Anatomic distribution and cancer potential of colonic polyps: An analysis of 7,000 polyps endoscopically removed. *Ann Surg* 190:679, 1979.

Silverberg E: Cancer of the colon and rectum: Statistical data. New York, American Cancer Society.

Silverberg SG: Locally malignant adenomatous polyps of the colon and rectum. *Surg Gynecol Obstet* 131:103, 1970.

Sivak MV Jr, Sullivan BH Jr, Weakley FL, et al: Colonoscopic polypectomy. *Dig Dis* 19(4), 1974.

Sivak MV Jr, Sullivan BH Jr, Rankin GB: Colonoscopy; a report of 644 cases and review of the literature. *Am J Surg* 128:351, 1974.

Skucas J, Cutcliff W, Fischer HW: Whole gut irrigation as a means of cleansing the colon. *Radiology* 121:303, 1976.

Smith LE: Fiberoptic colonoscopy: Complications of colonoscopy and polypectomy. *Dis Colon Rectum* 19:5, 1976.

Smith LE, Nivatvongs S: Complications in colonoscopy. *Dis Colon Rectum* 18:3, 1975.

Sobel HJ, Schwarz R, Marquet E: Light and electronmicroscope study of the origin of granular cell myoblastoma. *J Pathol* 109:101, 1973.

Soullard J, Potet F, Landrieu P: Les polyposes juveniles diffuses. *Arch Fr Mal Appar Dig* 61:391, 1972.

Spiro HM: *Clinical Gastroenterology*. London, MacMillan, 1970, vol II.

Spratt TSJ, Ackerman LV, Moyer CA: Relationship of polyps of the colon to colonic cancer. *Ann Surg* 148:682, 1958.

Swinton NW, Weakley FL: Complications of colotomy and colonoscopy. *Dis Colon Rectum* 6:50, 1963.

Sugarbaker PH, Vineyard GC: Snare polypectomy with the fiberoptic colonoscope. *Surg Gynecol Obstet* 138:581, 1974.

Sugarbaker P, Vineyard GC: Fiberoptic colonoscopy. A new look at old problems. *Am J Surg* 125:429, 1973.

Tanaka H, Sato Y, Uchida T: Peutz-Jeghers syndrome: One case and a survey of cases in Japan. *Clin All Round (Osaka)* 12:1411, 1963.

Teague RH, Salmon PR, Read AE: Fiberoptic examination of the colon: A review of 255 cases. *Gut* 14:139, 1973.

Turell R: Fiberoptic coloscope and sigmoidoscope. Preliminary report. *Am J Surg* 105:133, 1963.

Turell R: Fiberoptic sigmoidoscopes. *Am J Surg* 113:305, 1967.

Turell R: *Disease of Colon and Rectum*, ed 2. Philadelphia, WB Saunders, 1969, vol 1, p 359.

Turell R: *Diseases of the Colon and Ano Rectum*, ed 2. Philadelphia, WB Saunders, 1969, p 201.

Turnbull RB, Kyle K, Watson FR, et al: Cancer of the colon, in Maingot R (ed): *Abdominal Operations*, ed 6. New York, Appleton-Century-Crofts, 1974, p 2027.

Tuttle JP: *A Treatise on Diseases of the Anus, Rectum and Pelvic Colon*. New York, Appleton & Co, 1905.

Warwick RRG, Sumerling MD, Glimour HM, et al: Colonoscopy and double contrast barium enema examination in chronic ulcerative colitis. *Am J Roentgenol Radium Ther Nucl Med* 117:292, 1973.

Waye JD: Coloscopy. *Surg Clin N Am* 52(4): 1972.

Waye JD: The current status of flexible fiberoptic endoscopy. *Mt Sinai J Med* 42:21, 1975.

Waye JD: The role of colonoscopy in the differential diagnosis of inflammatory bowel disease. *Gastrointest Endosc* 23:150, 1977.

Welch EE: *Polypoid Lesions of the Gastrointestinal Tract*. Philadelphia, WB Saunders, 1964.

Welin S: Results of the Malmo technique of colon examination. *J Am Med Ass* 199:369, 1967.

Welin S: Newer diagnostic techniques. The superiority of double-contrast roentgenology. *Dis Colon Rectum* 17:13, 1974.

Wenzl JE, et al: Gastrointestinal polyposis with mucocutaneous pigmentation in children (Peutz-Jeghers syndrome). *Pediatrics* 28:655, 1961.

Williams C, Muto T: Examination of the whole colon with the fiberoptic colonoscope. *Gut* 13:322, 1972; *Br Med J* 3:278, 1972.

Williams CB: Diathermy-biopsy: A technique for the endoscopic management of small polyps. *Endoscopy* 5:215, 1973.

Williams CB: Coloscopy: A critical comment. *Acta Gastro-enterol Belg* 37:129, 1974.

Williams CB, Teague RM: Colonoscopy progress report. *Gut* 14:990, 1973.

Williams CB, Muto T, Rutter C: Removal of polyps with fiberoptic colonoscope: A new approach to colonic polypectomy. *Br Med J* 1:451, 1973.

Wolff WI, Shinya H: Colonfiberoscopy. *J Am Med Ass* 217:1509, 1971.

Wolff WI, Shinya H: Modern endoscopy of the alimentary tract. *Probl Surg* :50, Jan. 1974.

Wolff WI, Shinya H: Colonfiberoscopy: Diagnostic modality and therapeutic application. *Bull Soc Int Curr Chir* 5-6:525, 1971.

Wolff WI, Shinya H, Geffen A, et al: Colonfiberoscopy: A new and valuable diagnostic modality. *Am J Surg* 123:180, 1972.

Wolff WI, Shinya H: Colonfiberscopic management of colonic polyps. *Dis Colon Rectum* 16:87, 1973.

Wolff WI, Shinya H: A new approach to colonic polyps. *Ann Surg* 178:367, 1973.

Wolff WI, Shinya H: A new approach to the management of colonic polyps. *Adv Surg* 7:45, 1973.

Wolff WI, Shinya H: Earlier diagnosis of cancer of the colon through colonic endoscopy (colonoscopy). *Cancer (Philadelphia)* 34:912, 1974.

Wolff WI, Shinya H, Geffen A, et al: Colonofiberoscopy. *Am J Surg* 123:180, 1972.

Wolff WI, Shinya H: Modern endoscopy of the alimentary tract. *Curr Probl Surg* p 50, Jan, 1974.

Wolff WI, Shinya H, Geffen A, et al: Comparison of colonoscopy and the contrast enema in five hundred patients with colorectal disease. *Am J Surg* 129: 1975.

Wolff WI, Shinya H: Endoscopic polypectomy: Therapeutic and clinico-pathologic aspects. *Cancer (Philadelphia)* 36:683, 1975.

Wolff WI, Shinya H: Definitive treatment of malignant polyps of the colon. *Ann Surg* 182:516, 1975.

Wolff WI, Shinya H: The use of endoscopic polypectomy in improving survival in cancer of the colon. *Bull Soc Int Chir* 5: 1975.

Wolff WI, Grossman M, Shinya H: Angiodysplasia of the colon: Diagnosis and treatment. *Gastroenterology* 72:329, 1977.

Wolff WI, Shinya H: The impact of colonoscopy on the problem of colorectal cancer, in Ariel M (ed): *Progress in Clinical Cancer.* New York, Grune & Stratton, 1979, vol 7.

Woodward NW: Prevention of explosion while fulgurating polyps of the colon. *Dis Colon Rectum* 4:32, 1961.

Yamagata S, Oshiba S, Watanabe H: New fiberendoscope and its application to the colonic diseases, in *Proceedings of the 1st Congress of the International Society of Endoscopy*, Tokyo, 1966, p. 431.

Yamagata S, et al: Clinical experience of fibercolonoscope type VI. *Gastroenterol Endosc* II:219, 1969.

Zabeetakis MG: Flammability characteristics of combustible gases and vapors. U.S. Bureau of Mines, Bulletin 627: Methane, p 21; Hydrogen, p 89.

Zimmerman K: Detonation of intestinal gas by an electrosurgical unit. *South Med J* 52:605, 1959.

Index